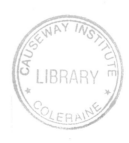
THE CANCER BOOK

A Guide to Understanding the Causes, Prevention, and Treatment of Cancer

GEOFFREY M. COOPER, Ph.D.
Professor of Pathology
Harvard Medical School
Dana-Farber Cancer Institute

JONES AND BARTLETT PUBLISHERS
Boston   London

Editorial, Sales, and Customer Service Offices
Jones and Bartlett Publishers
One Exeter Plaza
Boston, MA 02116
617-859-3900
1-800-832-0034

Jones and Bartlett Publishers International
7 Melrose Terrace
London W6 7RL
England

Library of Congress Cataloging-in-Publication Data
Cooper, Geoffrey M.
    The cancer book : a guide to understanding the causes, prevention, and treatment of cancer / Geoffrey M. Cooper.
        p.   cm.
    Includes bibliographical references and index.
    ISBN 0-86720-770-1
    1. Cancer--Popular works. I. Title.
RC263.C654   19931
616.99'4--dc20   93-16282
                                                                      CIP

The information presented in this book is accurate and current to the best of the author's knowledge. The author and the publisher, however, make no guarantee as to, and assume no responsibility for, the correctness, sufficiency, or completeness of such information or recommendations. The reader is advised to consult a physician regarding all aspects of individual health care.

Printed in the United States of America
97 96 95   10 9 8 7 6 5 4 3

To Dee and Ed

Contents

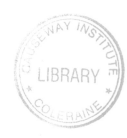

PART II

CAUSES OF CANCER   37

PART III

CANCER PREVENTION AND TREATMENT   97

PART IV

OVERVIEW OF MAJOR TYPES OF CANCER   155

12.   Leukemias and Lymphomas   157

13.   Childhood Solid Tumors   168

14.   Common Solid Tumors of Adults   174

PART V

PROSPECTS FOR THE FUTURE   195

15.   The War on Cancer—Progress and
Promises   197

Preface

Although cancer is one of our most common health problems, there are few sources of basic information about cancer available to the general public. Yet, this disease strikes one out of every three Americans, so many of us have a number of fundamental questions about it. What is cancer? How many different kinds are there? What causes cancer? Can it be prevented? How can cancer be treated, and how well do these treatments work? What is going on in cancer research? Will there ever be a cure for cancer? The answers to these questions are both of general interest, and—in all too many cases—of immediate practical consequence.

The Cancer Book is intended to meet the needs of readers wishing to obtain a broad understanding of the cancer problem. The book is written in nontechnical language with the goal of helping the reader understand the basic nature and causes of cancer, as well as the principles underlying current strategies for cancer prevention and treatment. It is hoped that *The Cancer Book* will provide an overview of, and perspective on, both the basic and practical aspects of cancer, including the background needed to understand continuing advances in our attempts to deal with this disease.

This book is derived from my recently published college textbook, *Elements of Human Cancer*, and a number of individuals have made critical contributions to both projects. My wife, Ann, was instrumental in encouraging me to write a general book on cancer, and patiently reviewed many drafts of the manuscript. *Elements of Human Cancer* was reviewed by a number of individuals who are experts in various aspects of cancer: Dr. Robert Bast (Duke Comprehensive Cancer Center), Dr. Dorothea Becker (University of Pittsburgh Cancer Center), Dr. Joseph Bertino (Memorial Sloan-Kettering Cancer Center), Dr. Charles Boone (National Cancer Institute), Dr. Hung Fan (University of California, Irvine), Dr. Florence Haseltine (National Institute of Child Health and Human Development), Dr. Carol McClure (University of California, Riverside), Dr. Paul Neiman (Fred Hutchinson Cancer Research Center), Dr. Albey Reiner (University of Massachusetts, Amherst), Dr. Machelle

Seibel (Faulkner Centre for Reproductive Medicine, Harvard Medical School), and Dr. Bert Vogelstein (The Johns Hopkins Oncology Center). I am grateful for their thoughtful comments and suggestions, which have been incorporated into the present book. In an effort to ensure that *The Cancer Book* would be clear to the general reader, it was also reviewed by three nonspecialists: Dortha Anderson, John Britton, and Ryan Kiessling. Their input was especially helpful in making the book understandable and accessible to readers without medical or scientific backgrounds. Finally, it is a pleasure to thank Don Jones, Paul Prindle, Joe Burns, Paula Carroll, and Judy Songdahl of Jones and Bartlett Publishers for their interest, support, and encouragement throughout the many stages of this project, and Helen Pultz for her editorial assistance.

PART I

The Nature of Cancer

Chapter 1

Basic Facts about Cancer

Cancer may be the most feared disease of our time. It is second only to heart disease as a leading cause of death in the United States, and it is estimated that one in every three Americans will develop cancer at some point in their lives. In spite of the major progress that has been made in cancer treatment, about half of patients with cancer ultimately die of their disease. Moreover, there is something intrinsically frightening about the very nature of cancer. Cancer results from abnormal growth of otherwise healthy cells. Cancer cells continue to grow and divide without restraint, eventually spreading throughout the body, interfering with the function of normal tissues and organs, and progressively leading to death. Some of the horror of cancer may be the feeling that a part of one's own body has revolted against the whole, leading to destruction from within.

WHAT IS CANCER?

Cancer is a disease fundamentally characterized by uncontrolled cell growth. There are many kinds of cancer; it is really a family of over one hundred different diseases. As is discussed later, the distinctions between the various kinds of cancer are of great practical importance, since they are treated differently and can have quite distinct outcomes for the patient. Not only are there numerous kinds of cancer, but individual cancers of the same type sometimes behave very differently from each other. For the patient and family members facing a diagnosis of cancer, it is critical to realize that the diagnosis is not a death sentence. Some patients with cancer can be readily cured. In other cases, life can be prolonged for many years by effective therapies.

In spite of this considerable diversity between individual cancers, the basic defect in all forms of cancer is the uncontrolled growth and division of cancer cells. Cells, the smallest living structures, are the fundamental units of which all living things are composed. The human body, for example, contains approximately 50 trillion individual cells, which make up tissues and organs such as the liver, heart, and brain. Each of these cells (which are less than 1/1000 inch in diameter) is specialized to perform one of the many individual tasks that the human body must accomplish daily. Thus, different types of cells are responsible for such diverse activities as digestion, movement, sight, and thought. Normally, all of these cells work together, in a coordinated manner, to serve the needs of the organism as a whole. As an analogy, consider a society (the body) made up of a large number of individuals (cells). Each individual performs specialized tasks, such as farming, building houses, or writing books, that, under ideal conditions, contribute to the common good.

Like the individuals that make up human societies, individual cells are capable of growth and reproduction, which occur by the division of one parent cell into two daughter cells. Importantly, however, the reproduction of individual cells is not an independent process. Instead, the growth and division of normal cells are carefully controlled to meet the needs of the whole organism.

Since the entire body originates from a single cell—the fertilized egg—there are obviously a great deal of cell growth and division during normal development. The behavior of individual cells is programmed as part of the overall developmental scheme, so that each cell grows and divides as required to form the tissues and organs of the developing embryo. In the adult, a few kinds of cells (such as nerve cells) are no longer capable of division, but most types of cells continue to divide as required to replace cells that have been lost due to cell injury or death. Skin cells, for example, are continually shed and must be replaced by cell division. Some types of cells, such as the blood-forming cells, those that line the intestine, and those that form hair, divide particularly rapidly throughout adult life. In these cases, frequent cell division is needed to replace mature cells that have short life spans. For example, nearly 1 trillion blood cells die each day in a normal adult, and these must be replaced by division of the blood-forming cells in the bone marrow. The system is carefully controlled so that the rate of division of the blood-forming cells precisely matches the rate of death of the mature blood cells. The division rates of other cell types are similarly regulated, so that the different tissues and organs are maintained at a functional, steady-state level in healthy adults.

This careful regulation of normal cell growth and division is lost in cancer cells. Cancer cells continue to grow and divide when they should not, apparently oblivious to the factors that control the growth and division of their normal counterparts. Cancer begins when a single cell begins to proliferate abnormally. This altered cell divides to form two abnormally proliferating cells, which in turn divide to form four abnormal cells, and so on (Fig. 1.1). Since each cancer cell divides to form two new cancer cells, the total number of cancer cells continues to increase

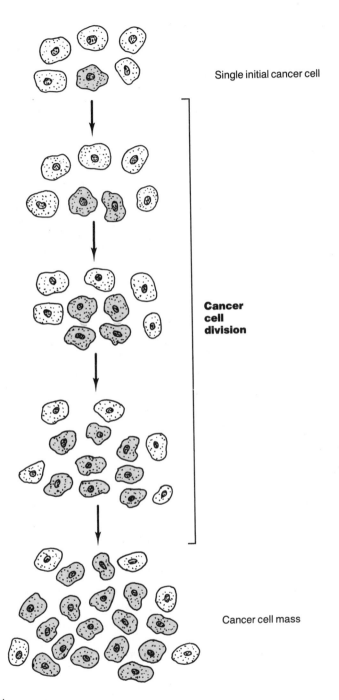

Single initial cancer cell

Cancer
cell
division

Cancer cell mass

Figure 1.1

Proliferation of cancer cells. Each cancer cell divides to form two new cancer cells so that the number of cancer cells doubles with each cell division.

rapidly. Thus, in this simple example, only twenty cell divisions result in the formation of about 1 million cancer cells from one abnormal cell. After another twenty cell divisions, the number of cancer cells in such a hypothetical tumor would be approximately 1 trillion—a number that would correspond to about one pound of tissue. Rapidly growing cells can divide as often as once a day, so that a single cancer cell dividing at this rate could develop, in a little over a month, to a tumor one pound in size (40 cell divisions = 40 days). The size of most tumors in the body does not increase this rapidly, however, and it usually takes several months or years for a cancer this large to develop. In addition, as will be discussed in later chapters, cancers actually develop in a much more gradual way, so that lengthy periods of time are generally required before an altered cell becomes a full-fledged cancer.

Overly simplistic though it may be, the above example illustrates the salient feature that is central to the understanding of cancer. Cancer is fundamentally a disease in which cell proliferation goes out of control. Consequently, these cells continue to grow and divide, yielding an ever increasing mass of more and more cancer cells. Unless checked, the cancer cells invade surrounding normal tissues, enter the circulation, and spread throughout the body, eventually interfering with the function of normal cells and leading to death of the patient.

THE CRITICAL QUESTION: IS IT BENIGN OR MALIGNANT?

The terminology used by physicians and scientists to describe different types of cancer is highly technical and often complicated. Some of this terminology will be discussed in later chapters, particularly with respect to the major types of cancer, which are described individually in Part IV. However, one issue is so critical to all aspects of dealing with the disease that it and the associated terminology need to be considered at this point—namely, the distinction between benign and malignant tumors.

A tumor, or neoplasm, is any abnormal growth of cells, which may be either benign or malignant. A benign tumor remains confined to its original location. It neither invades surrounding normal tissue nor spreads to distant body sites. A common skin wart is an example of a benign tumor. Since benign tumors remain localized to their site of origin, they can almost always be completely removed by surgery. Therefore, benign tumors are generally not life-threatening, except for those that occur in inoperable locations, such as some brain tumors.

In contrast, a malignant tumor is capable both of invading adjacent normal tissue and of spreading to other tissues and organs. Only malignant tumors are properly called cancers, and it is their ability to invade normal tissues and spread throughout the body, or metastasize, that makes cancer so dangerous. Once metastasis has occurred, cancer can no longer be successfully dealt with by localized treatment such as surgery. The ability of malignant tumors to invade and metastasize thus constitutes cancer's principal health hazard.

HOW FREQUENT IS CANCER?

It is estimated that approximately one out of every three Americans will develop cancer at some point during life. Currently, in spite of intensive research and some major advances in treatment, cancer claims the life of nearly one out of every four Americans (22%). Cancer is thus second only to heart disease, which is responsible for about 35 percent of deaths, as a cause of mortality in this country. Other causes of death, such as accidents, murders, and AIDS, each account for less than 5 percent of all deaths in the United States. About 1 million cases of cancer are diagnosed each year in the United States, and about 500,000 Americans die annually of the disease. Moreover, the number of cancer deaths continues to increase steadily. For example, approximately 514,000 Americans died of cancer in 1991. The corresponding number was approximately 510,000 in 1990, 502,000 in 1989, and 485,000 in 1988.

Although cancer is clearly a major affliction of contemporary society, this was not always the case. Cancer has been with us throughout the history of humanity, but has only become a leading cause of death within the last century. Prior to 1900, cancer was a comparatively rare disease that accounted for a relatively small percentage of deaths. At that time, most deaths were due to infectious diseases, such as influenza, pneumonia, and tuberculosis; and life expectancy was less than fifty years. Now, due both to general improvements in public health (such as sanitation, nutrition, and personal hygiene) and to development of vaccines and antibiotics, infectious diseases have been virtually eliminated as major causes of death. Consequently, life expectancy has increased to over seventy years, and the major causes of death have shifted to heart disease and cancer. The prevalence of cancer in current society is thus largely a consequence of the elimination of other diseases that constituted major killers in the past. The triumph of medical science against infectious disease has brought new health problems—cancer and heart disease—to the forefront of our present concerns.

THE DIFFERENT KINDS OF CANCER

There are over one hundred different kinds of cancer, which originate from different types of normal cells. As noted above, the terminology by which cancers are classified and named is complicated and will not be discussed in detail here. Most cancers fall into one of three main groups: carcinomas, sarcomas, and leukemias/lymphomas. Carcinomas, which constitute approximately 90 percent of all human cancers, arise from cells that cover the surface of the body (skin), line the internal organs (such as the lungs, stomach, and intestine), and form glands (such as the breast and prostate). Sarcomas, which are rare in humans, are cancers of connective tissues, such as muscle and bone. Leukemias and lymphomas, which constitute about 8 percent of all human cancers, arise from the blood-forming cells and cells of the immune system, respectively. Each of these main groups of cancers is further subdivided according to its site of origin (e.g., lung carcinoma) and a more detailed description of the type of cell involved.

Although there are many different kinds of cancer, only a few occur frequently. In fact, cancers of only eleven different sites account for about 80 percent of all cancers in the United States (Table 1.1). The most fre-

Table 1.1
MOST FREQUENT CANCERS IN THE UNITED STATES

Cancer Site	Cases per Year		Deaths per Year	
Lung	157,000	(15%)	142,000	(28%)
Colon/Rectum	155,000	(15%)	61,000	(12%)
Breast	151,000	(14%)	44,000	(9%)
Prostate	106,000	(10%)	30,000	(6%)
Bladder	49,000	(5%)	10,000	(2%)
Uterus	47,000	(5%)	10,000	(2%)
Lymphomas	43,000	(4%)	20,000	(4%)
Oral Cavity	31,000	(3%)	8,000	(2%)
Pancreas	28,000	(3%)	25,000	(5%)
Leukemias	28,000	(3%)	18,000	(4%)
Skin	28,000	(3%)	9,000	(2%)
	823,000	(79%)	377,000	(74%)
ALL SITES	1,040,000	(100%)	510,000	(100%)

Figures are for the year 1990. Nonmelanoma skin cancers (approximately 600,000 cases per year) and carcinomas of the uterine cervix diagnosed *in situ* (approximately 50,000 cases per year) are not included, since these cancers are readily curable. (From American Cancer Society, *Cancer Facts and Figures*, 1990.)

quent is skin cancer, which accounts for over 600,000 cases a year. However, the vast majority of skin cancers are highly curable and are therefore not included in Table 1.1. The next four most common are cancers of the lung, the colon and rectum, the breast, and the prostate. Together, these four account for over half of all cancer cases. Lung cancer is the most frequent lethal cancer, with approximately 157,000 cases per year; it accounts for over one-fourth of all cancer deaths. About one-half of all cancer deaths are caused by three kinds of cancer—those of the lung, the breast, and the colon and rectum.

The frequency of many kinds of cancer has remained relatively constant over the last fifty years, but some have changed significantly (Fig. 1.2). The most striking change is in the frequency of lung cancer, which has increased more than ten-fold since 1930. This continuing increase in the frequency of lung cancer accounts for the steady rise in the overall incidence of cancer in the United States. As will be discussed more fully

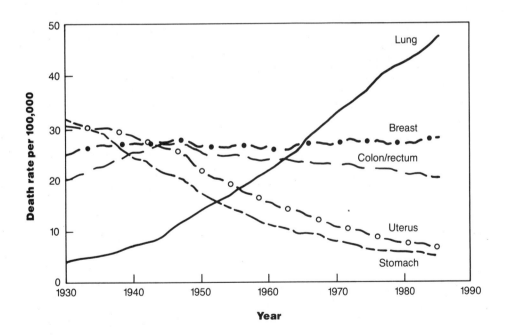

Figure 1.2

Death rates for representative cancers since 1930. Annual death rates are shown for the United States population. Rates for lung, colon/rectum, and stomach cancers are for both sexes. Rates for cancers of the breast and uterus (both cervix and endometrium) are for women only. (From American Cancer Society, *Cancer Facts and Figures*, 1990.)

in chapter 4, the rise in lung cancer incidence is directly attributable to increased use of tobacco, particularly cigarette smoking. It follows that lung cancer could be effectively prevented by cessation of tobacco use, which would eliminate a major fraction of cancer deaths.

In contrast to the increasing mortality from lung cancer, there have been significant decreases in deaths from cancers of the stomach and uterine cervix (Fig. 1.2). In 1930, stomach cancer was the most common cause of cancer death, and cervical cancer was second. However, the incidence of stomach cancer has now declined more than five-fold. The reason for this substantial decrease in stomach cancer is probably related to changes in dietary practices, as discussed further in chapters 4 and 8. Interestingly, the incidence of stomach cancer remains very high in other countries. For example, stomach cancer is the most common cancer in Japan, with an incidence about eight times higher than in the United States. As discussed in detail in chapter 4, such differences between countries suggest the importance of environmental factors—for example, differences in diet between Japan and the United States—as causes of cancer.

Whereas the decline in mortality from stomach cancer is due to a decreased incidence of the disease, the decline in mortality from cervical cancer is due, at least in part, to improved diagnosis and treatment. More specifically, cancer of the uterine cervix can be diagnosed at an early stage by microscopic examination of a sample of cells from the cervix, which can readily be obtained as part of a routine physical examination. This is the Pap test, named after its originator, George Papanicolau. Abnormal cervical cells can be reliably identified in such samples, allowing detection of this cancer at an early stage of the disease when it can be effectively and easily treated. Over 50,000 cases of cervical cancer are diagnosed and cured in this way each year in the United States. The Pap test is thus the classic success story of an early screening test, which will be discussed further in chapter 9.

CANCER AND AGE

Cancer can occur at any age, but it becomes much more common as we grow older. This is illustrated in Fig. 1.3 for the three most common cancers, those of the lung, the breast, and the colon and rectum. The incidence of colon and rectum cancer, for example, increases more than ten-fold between the ages of thirty and fifty, and another ten-fold between fifty and seventy. Such dramatic increases in cancer incidence with age are, of course, directly related to the prevalence of cancer in modern society. As discussed above, elimination of infectious diseases resulted in a substantial increase in the average life span, leading to a larger fraction

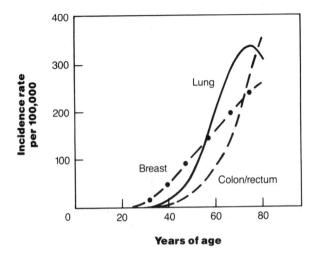

Figure 1.3

Relation of cancer incidence to age. Annual incidence rates are shown for both sexes in the United States. (Data are plotted from National Cancer Institute, *Cancer Statistics Review*, 1989.)

of older individuals, and a correspondingly greater incidence of cancer, in our population.

The increasing incidence of cancer with age reflects a fundamental feature of the biology of cancer cells. As will be discussed further in later chapters, the conversion of a normal cell to a cancer cell does not occur as a single one-step event. Rather, the loss of growth control that characterizes cancer cells is the end result of accumulated mutations in multiple different genes regulating normal cell growth. Development of cancer thus involves a series of progressive changes which gradually convert a normal cell into one that has lost control of its proliferation. Many years are required to accumulate the multiple abnormalities needed to generate most cancer cells, so the majority of cancers develop relatively late in life.

Not all cancers, however, are confined to advancing age. Indeed, the most tragic cancers are those of childhood. Fortunately, cancer is comparatively rare in children. Of the approximately 1 million cases of cancer diagnosed yearly in the United States, less than 8000 affect children. Nonetheless, cancer is responsible for about 10 percent of deaths in children under age fifteen, making it second only to accidents (which cause about 40% of childhood deaths) as a leading cause of childhood mortality. The common adult cancers are rare in children. Instead, cancers of the blood and immune systems, leukemias and lymphomas, account for about half of all childhood cancers. The other kinds of cancers that are common in children, including cancers of the brain, nervous system, bone, and kidney, are rare in adults.

TREATMENT OF CANCER

As will be discussed in detail in chapter 10, cancer is treated by surgery, radiation, and chemotherapy. The success of these treatments varies considerably according to the kind of cancer and how early it is detected. As noted above, the common skin cancers and cancer of the uterine cervix can be detected at very early stages, at which time they can be readily cured. As will be discussed in later chapters, early detection and treatment of breast and of colon and rectum cancers are also of major importance to the outcome of these diseases.

The success of treatment of most cancers is usually measured as the fraction of patients who survive for five years without evidence of disease. Most patients surviving this long can be considered to have been cured of their cancer, although in some cases the cancer may recur even after this time.

The overall five-year survival rate for all cancers is now about 50 percent, and survival rates for some of the common adult cancers are illustrated in Fig. 1.4. The most common cancer of adults, lung cancer, is difficult to detect before the disease has reached an advanced stage, and only about 10 percent of patients with lung cancer survive five years after diagnosis. The five-year survival rates for the other major adult cancers are, however, more encouraging: approximately 75 percent for breast cancer, 70 percent for prostate cancer, and 50 percent for colon and rectum cancer. These survival rates are substantially influenced by the time at which the cancer is detected and treatment is initiated. For example, the five-year survival rate for breast cancer is over 90 percent if the cancer is detected early, but declines to only about 20 percent if the cancer has progressed to an advanced stage and spread (metastasized) to distant body sites by the time of diagnosis. At the other extreme is pancreatic cancer, which is not usually detected until an advanced stage and is associated with a five-year survival rate of only 3 percent.

The development of effective therapies for some of the childhood leukemias and lymphomas has been a major, and particularly gratifying, advance in cancer treatment. Chemotherapy now leads to cures for up to 75 percent of children with acute lymphocytic leukemia, the most common childhood cancer. In contrast, this disease was fatal for more than 95 percent of the children diagnosed in 1960. Chemotherapy for lymphomas has also been highly effective, with survival rates of up to 90 percent for Hodgkin's disease and 60 percent for non-Hodgkin's

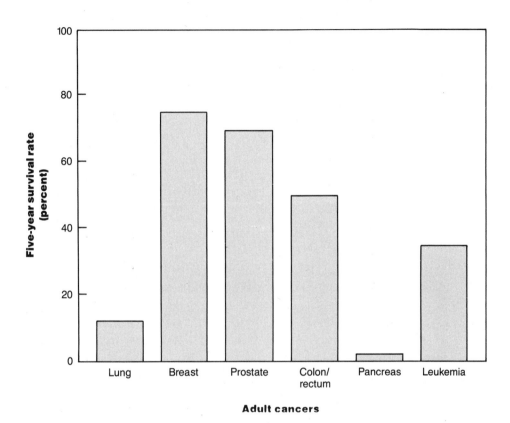

Figure 1.4

Survival rates for representative adult cancers. Five-year survival rates for all stages of the indicated cancers are shown for the United States. (From American Cancer Society, *Cancer Facts and Figures,* 1990.)

lymphomas. Survival rates for other childhood cancers are about 50 percent for bone, brain, and nervous system cancers and over 80 percent for kidney cancer (Wilms' tumor).

Substantial advances in the treatment of cancer have clearly been made, and the diagnosis of cancer is no longer a hopeless one. In addition, in many cases, appropriate therapy can prolong life for many years even if a cure is not achieved. Nonetheless, the fact remains that many patients with cancer eventually die of their disease, so current treatments are ultimately unsuccessful. Moreover, the survival rates for the most common adult cancers (lung, breast, and colon/rectum) have improved only slightly over the last thirty years.

The prospect of a cure for cancer, in the way that penicillin is a cure for many bacterial infections, remains a distant hope. The difficulty lies in the nature of cancer compared to the infectious diseases. Penicillin is an effective antibiotic because it kills the bacteria causing disease without damaging the normal cells of the body. This works because there are major differences between bacterial cells and our own. In particular, penicillin prevents synthesis of the bacterial cell wall. Since animal cells do not have a cell wall, the normal cells of the body are unaffected by penicillin. The success of antibiotics is thus based on fundamental differences between bacteria and human cells.

Cancer, on the other hand, is due to uncontrolled growth of some of the cells of our own bodies. There are, therefore, no readily apparent targets (like the bacterial cell wall) for a "magic bullet" against cancer. As will be discussed in subsequent chapters, most of the drugs currently used in cancer therapy are directed against *all* rapidly dividing cells. They consequently affect not only cancer cells but also some normal cells, particularly those that line the intestine, form hair, and form blood cells. Since such drugs kill normal cells in addition to cancer cells, they are quite toxic to the patient, and this toxicity severely limits their effectiveness. As a result, much of the present research on cancer is devoted to understanding the mechanisms that control normal cell division and to elucidating the abnormalities in cancer cells that result in their unregulated growth. The long range hope is that understanding the basis of normal and abnormal cell growth will eventually lead to new strategies for selectively blocking the growth and division of cancer cells.

SUMMARY

Cancer is second only to heart disease as the leading cause of death in the United States, and is expected to affect approximately one out of every three Americans. Although there are many different kinds of cancer, they all have a common fundamental basis: abnormal growth and division of cancer cells, which eventually spread through the body, invading and interfering with the function of normal tissues and organs. Cancer is thus a disease in which a cancer cell fails to respond to the controls that regulate normal cell growth and division. Such loss of growth control usually requires the accumulation of mutations in multiple different cellular regulatory genes, so most cancers develop late in life. Substantial progress has been made in the treatment of cancer, but in many cases current therapies ultimately fail, and about 50 percent of patients with cancer eventually die of their disease. Since cancer cells closely resemble normal cells, the fundamental problem in cancer treatment is selectively interfering with the growth of cancer cells without adverse side effects on the patient.

Chapter 2
The Development of Cancer

As discussed in the preceding chapter, cancer results from the uncontrolled growth of abnormal cells. Importantly, the development of cancer is a gradual process, one in which cancer cells become increasingly malignant and more rapidly dividing over time. This progressive nature of cancer development is of considerable practical significance, since it means that cancers diagnosed at an early stage can be treated more successfully than those that are advanced. The current approaches to early detection of cancer, and their potential impact on reducing cancer mortality, will be considered in chapter 9. This chapter discusses the ways in which cancers develop, invade normal tissue, and ultimately metastasize or spread throughout the body. The extent of tumor progression at the time of diagnosis determines the clinical stage of each individual cancer, thereby providing critical information with respect to prognosis and treatment.

TUMOR INITIATION AND PROGRESSION: THE EVOLUTION OF CANCER

A fundamental feature of the development of cancer, already noted in chapter 1, is that a tumor develops from only a single cell that begins to proliferate abnormally. Thus, all of the cells in a tumor arise from the growth and division of the same cell of origin. Since tumor cells inevitably divide to form more tumor cells, the continued proliferation of a single abnormal cell gives rise to a continually increasing tumor cell population.

In spite of the fact that tumors originate from single cells, it is important to realize that the first cell that begins to divide abnormally has not yet acquired all of the malignant characteristics of a full-blown cancer cell. On the contrary, normal cells become converted to cancer cells, not in a single step, but through a series of changes that lead to increasingly abnormal cell growth, culminating in malignancy. As noted in chapter 1, most cancers are much more frequent in older people than in younger ones. This increasing incidence of cancer with age is a reflection of the fact that the generation of a cancer cell is a stepwise process, requiring the accumulation of multiple alterations over time.

The development of cancer is thus viewed as a multistep process involving the accumulation of damage to critical genes that regulate cell growth, followed by the proliferation of ever more rapidly growing tumor cells with increasing invasiveness and metastatic potential (Fig. 2.1). The first step in the development of cancer is the result of a genetic alteration, or mutation, that affects a critical growth-regulatory gene in a single cell of the body. The next step is abnormal proliferation of that mutated cell, which leads to formation of an actively growing tumor cell population. However, this is not the end of the story. Tumor progression continues as additional mutations occur within cells of this proliferating population. These mutations may have a variety of effects on the cells, but, eventually, one will result in more rapid cell growth. Because of their increased growth potential, the descendants of a cell bearing such a mutation enjoy a selective advantage and outgrow the other cells in the tumor. When this occurs, a new population of tumor cells with increased proliferative potential becomes dominant, taking over the initial tumor cell population. This process of mutation and selection is repeated multiple times during tumor progression, resulting in the formation of more and more rapidly growing tumor cells. As will be discussed further in chapter 3, the genetic material of cancer cells may undergo more frequent alterations than that of normal cells, and this genetic instability could accelerate mutation and selection during tumor development. Tumor progression is thus viewed as a series of steps, each of which involves selection for more aggressive tumor cells with increased proliferative capacity, invasiveness, and metastatic potential. For many cancers, it has been estimated that four to six such steps are required for the development of a malignant tumor.

Colon cancer is a good example of the multistep development of a common human malignancy (Fig. 2.2). The earliest stage in tumor development, prior to formation of an actual tumor mass, is increased proliferation of some of the cells lining the colon. One of the cells within this rapidly dividing cell population is then thought to give rise to a small benign tumor, designated a small adenoma in Fig. 2.2. Further tumor progression results in the formation of adenomas (polyps) of increasing size and growth potential. Eventually, some of the adenoma cells begin to invade the underlying tissues of the colon wall. Such invasion is the hallmark of malignancy, so at this point the benign adenoma has progressed into a malignant carcinoma, or cancer. This is followed by the continuing spread of the cancer cells through the surrounding normal tissue and metastasis of the tumor to distant body sites.

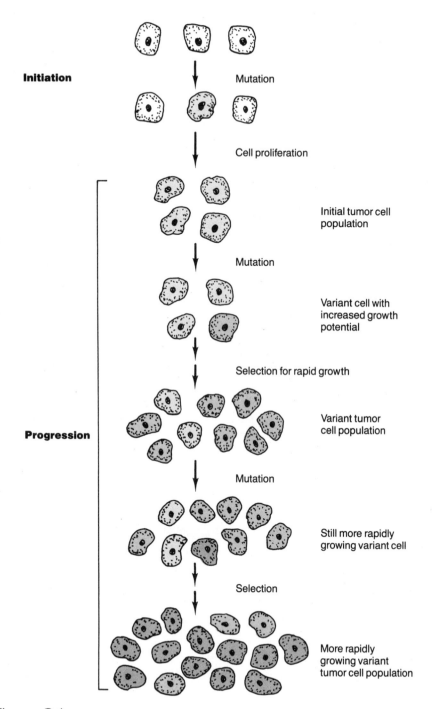

Initiation

Mutation

Cell proliferation

Initial tumor cell population

Mutation

Variant cell with increased growth potential

Selection for rapid growth

Progression

Variant tumor cell population

Mutation

Still more rapidly growing variant cell

Selection

More rapidly growing variant tumor cell population

Figure 2.1

Tumor development. A cancer develops through a series of steps, each of which involves mutation and selection for more rapidly growing cells within the tumor cell population.

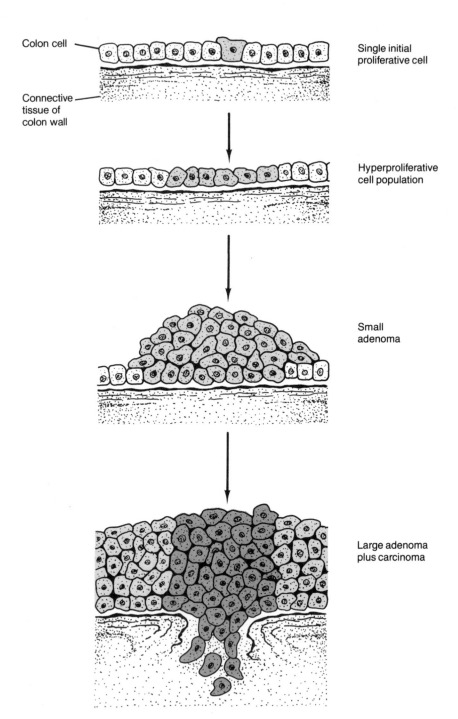

Colon cell

Connective tissue of colon wall

Single initial proliferative cell

Hyperproliferative cell population

Small adenoma

Large adenoma plus carcinoma

Figure 2.2

Development of colon/rectum carcinomas. A single altered cell gives rise to a hyperprolif-erative cell population, which progresses first to benign adenomas of increasing size and then to malignant carcinoma.

INVASION AND METASTASIS: THE CRITICAL
STEPS IN TUMOR DEVELOPMENT

The ability of malignant neoplasms to spread throughout the body rather than remaining confined to their site of origin is responsible for most cancer deaths. Benign tumors and carcinomas *in situ*—small tumors that have not yet invaded adjacent normal tissues—can be readily cured by localized surgical procedures. Once invasion of surrounding normal tissue has occurred, however, the effectiveness of surgery depends on removing all of the tissue that contains cancer cells. Finally, once the cancer has metastasized to distant body sites, surgery is no longer effective alone; it must be combined with chemotherapy to treat the disseminated disease. As noted in chapter 1, the common skin cancers (basal and squamous cell carcinomas) are highly curable because they only rarely metastasize. Likewise, the Pap test has been effective at reducing mortality from cervical cancer because it allows detection of carcinoma of the uterine cervix *in situ,* at which stage simple curative treatment is possible. For other cancers, however, metastasis has occurred by the time of diagnosis in more than 50 percent of patients.

The first step in progression from carcinoma *in situ* to metastatic carcinoma is invasion of the tumor cells into underlying normal tissue (*Fig. 2.3*). The cancer cells then continue to proliferate and spread through the normal tissue surrounding the site of the primary tumor. In some cases, the cancer cells can spread directly to adjacent organs. For example, colon carcinomas can penetrate through the wall of the colon and directly invade neighboring organs such as the bladder or small intestine. Most important, however, is entry of the tumor cells into the blood and lymphatic systems, since these are the major routes of tumor metastasis. Once a tumor has invaded normal tissue surrounding its site of origin, the cancer cells can penetrate blood and lymphatic vessels, allowing them to be carried throughout the body.

The circulatory system carries blood from the heart to all tissues of the body through the arteries, and then returns it back to the heart through the veins. Tumor cells can enter the circulatory system by invading capillaries, the small vessels in tissues through which oxygen and nutrients in fresh blood are exchanged for carbon dioxide and waste products. Once in the circulatory system, the cancer cells can be carried to any site in the body. They can then initiate growth in a new organ by again penetrating through the capillaries and invading the adjacent tissue. Many tumors metastasize most frequently to the organ that the tumor cells reach first via the circulatory system. For example, colon cancers often metastasize to the liver—the site to which the tumor cells are directly carried from

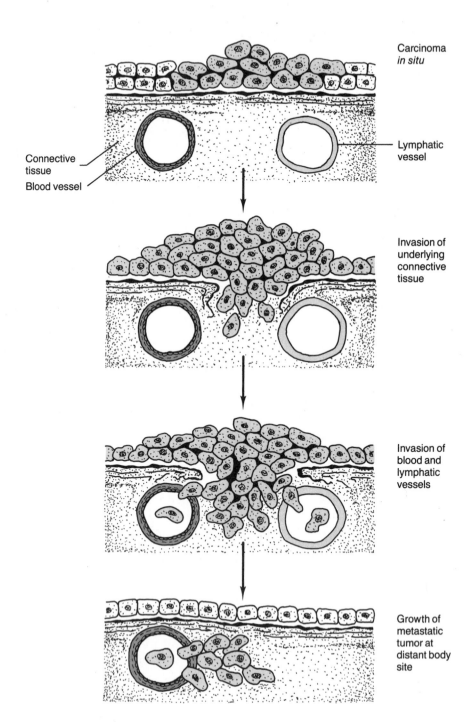

Carcinoma *in situ*

Connective tissue

Blood vessel

Lymphatic vessel

Invasion of underlying connective tissue

Invasion of blood and lymphatic vessels

Growth of metastatic tumor at distant body site

the colon by the circulatory system. In the liver, the tumor cells reach a network of capillaries through which they can leave the circulatory system and establish a new metastatic growth.

The lymphatic system (Fig. 2.4) is a drainage system through which fluid from tissues is carried back to the circulatory system. During this process, lymphatic fluid passes through a series of lymph nodes, which are small masses of tissue containing lymphocytes. Lymphocytes, the principal cells of the immune system, are also carried throughout the body in the lymphatic fluid and blood. The lymphatic system thus plays a major role in the body's defense against infection. In addition, as discussed below, it appears that lymphocytes can recognize and attack at least some cancer cells, thereby providing a natural defense mechanism against cancer development.

Cancer cells can invade lymphatic vessels in tissues in the same way they invade capillaries. Via the lymphatic system, they can spread throughout the body and enter the circulatory system as discussed above. Since metastasis via the lymphatic system results in the deposition of cancer cells in the lymph nodes, the extent to which a tumor has spread is frequently estimated by examining lymph nodes in the area of the tumor for the presence of cancer cells.

It is important to realize that entry of a cancer cell into the circulatory or lymphatic system is only the first step in metastasis of a tumor to a distant site. In order to successfully establish a metastatic growth, the cancer cells must first survive a turbulent journey through the circulatory system and evade recognition and destruction by the immune system. They then must attach to and penetrate the walls of blood vessels in order to initiate a new growth at a distant site. These factors represent formidable barriers to metastasis, and the vast majority of tumor cells that enter the circulation are eliminated. In fact, it is estimated that less than one in 10,000 successfully establish a metastatic tumor. However, since rapidly growing tumors can shed millions of cells into the circulation daily, metastasis is the inevitable result of the progression of malignant neoplasms.

← Figure 2.3

Invasion and metastasis. Cancer cells first invade underlying normal tissue and eventually reach and penetrate blood and lymphatic vessels. The cancer cells can then be carried throughout the body, leading to the establishment of metastatic tumors at distant body sites.

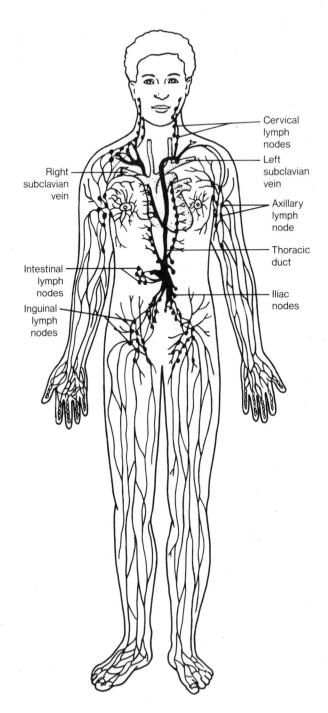

Cervical
lymph
nodes

Left
subclavian
vein

Right
subclavian
vein

Axillary
lymph
node

Thoracic
duct

Intestinal
lymph
nodes

Iliac
nodes

Inguinal
lymph
nodes

Figure 2.4

The lymphatic system.

THE IMMUNE SYSTEM: A NATURAL
DEFENSE AGAINST CANCER

As noted above, the immune system, the body's natural defense against infections, also appears capable of recognizing and eliminating at least some cancer cells, thus providing a natural protection against the development and spread of cancer. The cells of the immune system, lymphocytes, are formed in the bone marrow and then migrate to the lymphatic system, which includes the lymph nodes and spleen in addition to the thymus, tonsils, and adenoids. Lymphocytes are specialized to recognize and eliminate substances that are foreign to the body. Thus, they function as the body's surveillance system, geared to detect and repel "foreign invaders."

A principal function of the immune system is to provide protection against infectious agents, such as viruses and bacteria. In addition, lymphocytes can react against other human cells that are recognized as foreign or abnormal. All cells carry a variety of chemical markers on their surfaces. These cell-surface markers are recognized by the immune system, which can thus distinguish "self" from "nonself." If lymphocytes encounter cells that display nonself markers, an immune response against these foreign cells is mounted. For example, organ (e.g., kidney) transplants may be rejected if the immune system of the recipient recognizes the donor organ as foreign. To avoid such immune rejection, the physician performing a transplant makes sure that the cells of the donor and recipient are as similar as possible—ideally from identical twins. In addition, drugs are usually used to suppress the activity of the recipient's immune system until the transplanted organ has had an opportunity to establish itself.

Likewise the immune system is capable of recognizing and reacting against cancer cells. When normal cells become converted to cancer cells, they frequently display altered surface markers that are recognized as nonself. In such cases, the cancer cells may be attacked and eliminated by the resulting immune response. The effectiveness of the immune system in this regard is illustrated by the fact that individuals lacking normal immune function (such as AIDS patients) suffer a high incidence of several types of cancer. Unfortunately, however, cancer occurs all too frequently in otherwise normal individuals, so it is painfully obvious that many cancers manage to evade this defense mechanism. Nonetheless, as discussed in chapter 10, it may be possible to bolster the activity of the immune system against cancer cells, thereby providing a natural approach to cancer treatment.

CLINICAL STAGING OF CANCER

The extent of tumor progression at the time of diagnosis is of critical importance to prognosis and formulation of a plan of treatment. The degree to which cancers have progressed is generally described by clinical staging, with different systems frequently used to describe different kinds of tumors. However, the use of multiple staging systems, in which the same aspects of tumor progression are described in different ways, has created unnecessary complications of nomenclature. An alternative unified staging system, the TNM system, has been developed by the International Union Against Cancer and the American Joint Committee on Cancer. In this system, which is applicable to many different kinds of cancer, the extent of disease is described in terms of three considerations: T, the condition of the primary tumor; N, the extent of lymph node involvement; and M, the extent of distant metastases.

As an example, the staging of colon and rectum cancer by the TNM system is illustrated in Table 2.1. This indicates carcinoma *in situ*, and T1 through T4 indicate primary tumors characterized by increasing size and degrees of invasion of surrounding tissues.

N0 indicates that the lymph nodes in the area of the tumor appear free of cancer cells, whereas N1, N2, and N3 indicate increasing extents of lymph node involvement. M0 indicates the absence of detectable metastases to distant organs, while M1 indicates their presence. Unfortunately, many M0 patients have small metastatic lesions that are not detectable at the time of diagnosis. The likelihood of such small metastases is greater for patients with larger or more invasive tumors—increasing grades of T—or with lymph node involvement—increasing N. Hence, T and N grading is important in deciding on a plan of treatment following surgery.

The significance of tumor staging to prognosis and treatment is also readily illustrated for colon and rectum cancer. The five-year survival rate after surgery is greater than 90 percent for patients with T1N0M0 or T2N0M0 stage colon cancer, about 80 percent for T3N0M0 stage, and 60 to 70 percent for T4N0M0 stage. Prognosis after surgery is significantly poorer if there is lymph node involvement. For example, five-year survival rates after surgery are approximately 50 percent for T3N1M0 stage colon cancer and approximately 40 percent for T4N1M0 stage. In addition to surgery, further treatment with radiation and/or chemotherapy appears advantageous for patients with more advanced primary tumors (T3 or T4) or with lymph node involvement (N1 or N2). Patients with detectable metastatic disease (M1 stage) are usually no longer curable, although appropriate treatment can significantly prolong and enhance the quality of life.

TABLE 2.1
STAGING OF COLON AND RECTUM CANCER

Classification	Description
Primary Tumor	
Tis	Carcinoma *in situ*
T1	Invasion into submucosa layer of colon wall
T2	Invasion through submucosa into underlying muscular layer
T3	Invasion through muscular layer
T4	Invasion into peritoneal cavity and adjacent organs
Regional Lymph Nodes	
N0	Regional lymph nodes free of tumor
N1	1–3 positive nodes
N2	4 or more positive nodes
N3	Positive nodes on major vascular trunk
Distant Metastases	
M0	No distant metastases
M1	Distant metastases present

SUMMARY

Cancers originate with the abnormal growth and division of single mutated cells. The development of cancer, however, is a complex multistep process in which malignant cells gradually evolve as a result of a series of additional mutations. Tumor progression thus involves the accumulation of multiple mutations, leading to the formation of more rapidly growing and increasingly malignant cells within the tumor population. Eventually tumor progression leads to the development of metastatic cancers, which evade the immune system and spread to distant body sites. The extent of tumor progression at the time of diagnosis, described by clinical staging, is therefore a critical determinant of prognosis and treatment.

Chapter 3

How Cancer Cells Differ from Normal Cells

Since cancer results from the uncontrolled growth and division of abnormal cells, a major goal of many scientists has been to understand why cancer cells behave abnormally to begin with. If we understood what goes wrong in cancer cells, perhaps it would be possible to develop more effective means to either prevent or treat the disease. Ideally, strategies for prevention or treatment might be based on differences between cancer cells and the normal cells of our bodies, leading to the development of drugs that would specifically attack cancer cells with minimal damage to normal cells and tissues. While we are still far from achieving this goal, a great deal of progress has been made in understanding the basis for the unregulated growth of cancer cells. This chapter therefore discusses some of the ways in which cancer cells differ from their normal counterparts, and how these abnormalities in cancer cells relate to the progressive growth and spread of malignant tumors.

CONTROL OF NORMAL CELL BEHAVIOR

As discussed in chapter 1, cells are the building blocks of which all living things are composed. The human body consists of about 50 trillion individual cells, all of which normally function in a closely coordinated manner so that their individual activities meet the needs of the body as a whole. Thus, the behavior of each cell is carefully regulated to ensure that it functions as part of an integrated unit, not as an independent entity. In this sense, the body is a tightly controlled socialistic society in which the self-interest of each cell is subjugated to the collective need. The breakdown of this critical regulatory system leads to uncontrolled growth of a renegade cell, eventually resulting in the development of cancer.

All cells consist of two major parts: the nucleus and the cytoplasm (Fig. 3.1). Pursuing the analogy of a cell as an individual, the nucleus is

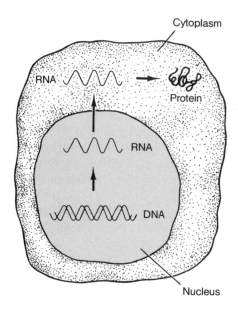

Cytoplasm

RNA

Protein

RNA

DNA

Nucleus

Figure 3.1

The organization of a cell. Cells consist of two major compartments, the cytoplasm and the nucleus. The nucleus contains the genetic material (DNA). Genes are expressed by being copied into RNA, which is transported to the cytoplasm where it directs synthesis of the specified protein. The protein then carries out the particular task directed by the gene in question.

the cell's brain, serving as the information center responsible for directing cell behavior. It contains the cell's genetic material (DNA), which can be viewed as a blueprint providing the specifications for all of the cell's activities. The complete genetic material of all human beings (the human genome) consists of about 100,000 individual genes, each of which codes for the synthesis of a specific protein. The information contained in each gene is expressed by being copied into RNA, which then directs synthesis of the specified protein in the cytoplasm of the cell. The protein is the active product of the gene, which is responsible for execution of the specific task directed by the gene in question.

The genetic material of each individual is assembled at the time of fertilization. Each gene is present in two copies, one derived from the egg and the other from the sperm. The genome of each individual contains all of the information needed to direct the development of a complete new human being from only a single cell, the fertilized egg. The development of the human mind and body from such seemingly humble beginnings is truly a marvel of biology.

Two distinct kinds of processes must take place during the development of each person: cell division and cell differentiation. Cell division generates the 50 trillion cells that make up an adult human. Cell differentiation is the specialization of these cells: some function as nerve cells, some as liver cells, some as muscle cells, and so forth. Both cell division and cell differentiation must be carefully regulated and coordinated in order for normal growth and development to take place.

In spite of the fact that different kinds of cells (e.g., nerve cells and muscle cells) perform very different functions, all the cells of each person contain the same genes. Each time a cell divides, the entire genome is replicated and passed on to each new cell. The reason that different kinds of cells behave differently is not that they contain different genes, but because only some genes are actually expressed in each cell type, resulting in the synthesis of proteins that specifically determine cell function. Thus, a muscle cell uniquely expresses particular genes that make it behave as a muscle cell, while a nerve cell expresses other genes that make it behave as a nerve cell. The specialization of cells to perform the many tasks required by the body is thus determined by which genes are expressed in each type of cell.

Cell growth and division are similarly controlled by gene expression. The expression of some genes stimulates a cell to grow and divide, whereas the expression of other genes inhibits cell division. The overall behavior of each of our cells—that is, their function as well as their growth and division—is therefore determined by the carefully regulated expression of the approximately 100,000 genes inherited by each human being. And it is mutations in some of these genes that can lead to inappropriate cell growth, resulting in the development of cancer.

Since the behavior of each cell is normally controlled to meet the needs of the entire body, it is apparent that all cells must have some means of knowing what is going on around them. A cell must be capable of sensing signals from its environment and responding appropriately, altering its growth or function to meet whatever physiological needs may arise. Such signals often come in the form of proteins or other chemicals, such as steroid hormones, which are secreted by one cell in order to communicate with another. For example, skin cells are normally stimulated to divide as needed to repair damage from a cut or wound. One element of this signaling system is a protein called platelet-derived growth factor or PDGF. PDGF is released from blood platelets during blood clotting. It then signals skin cells in the neighborhood of a cut to grow and divide in order to repair the damage.

A number of other hormones and growth factors, like PDGF, either stimulate or inhibit the division of appropriate types of cells as required to meet other physiological needs. The steroid hormone estrogen is a good example. Estrogen is normally produced by the ovaries during each menstrual cycle. It acts to stimulate division of the endometrial cells lining the uterus, thereby preparing it to receive an embryo in the event of pregnancy.

In addition to responding to growth factors and hormones, cells also respond to direct contact with their neighbors. Such direct interactions between cells are particularly important in determining the basic shape of the body, and it is critically important that different types of cells interact correctly with each other during development. For example, the formation of an arm requires the appropriately coordinated growth and arrangement of several different types of cells, including those forming muscles, bone, nerves, blood vessels, and skin.

In order to function correctly, then, each cell must be capable of sensing and responding appropriately to a variety of different signals from its environment, just as each individual needs to interact with other members of his or her society. Each cell therefore comes equipped with a battery of sensing devices, usually present on the cell's outer surface. When an appropriate signal is received at the cell surface, it sets off a series of chemical reactions within the cell. These reactions serve to transmit a signal from the surface to the cell nucleus, much as the nerves of our bodies transmit signals from our eyes or skin to our brains. Within the cell nucleus, the signal initiated at the cell surface acts to change the expression of specific genes, leading to appropriate alterations in cell behavior.

A good example is once again the behavior of skin cells in repairing damage resulting from a cut (Fig. 3.2). When blood clots, the growth factor PDGF is released from blood platelets. PDGF then interacts with a specific receptor on the surface of skin cells. This stimulates the receptor to transmit signals to the nucleus, leading to expression of genes that trigger cell division. The skin cells therefore begin to proliferate and

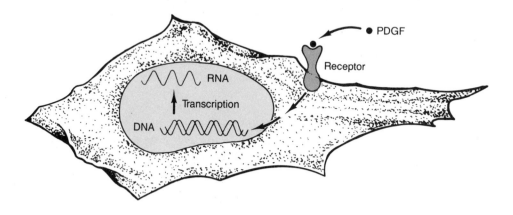

Figure 3.2

Response of a cell to platelet-derived growth factor (PDGF). PDGF is released during blood clotting and then binds to a specific receptor on the surface of skin cells. This initiates a series of reactions within the cell that transmit a signal to the nucleus, ultimately resulting in expression of genes that trigger cell division.

continue to divide until the cut is healed. Equally importantly, the cells also respond to signals (such as contact with their neighbors) that inhibit further cell division once the damage is repaired. Thus, skin cells are stimulated to grow and divide in a controlled manner, as required to meet the body's need to heal a wound.

ABNORMAL GROWTH OF CANCER CELLS

The basic defect in cancer cells is that they grow and divide in an uncontrolled fashion, rather than being regulated by the start and stop signals that control normal cell division. Cancer cells do not require appropriate stimulatory signals before dividing, and they fail to respond to the signals that inhibit division of normal cells. The characteristic unregulated proliferation of cancer cells results from a number of abnormalities that distinguish them from their normal counterparts.

As discussed above, normal cells only proliferate when stimulated by an appropriate growth factor. Such growth factors are typically produced by one type of cell in order to signal the division of a different cell type in response to a particular physiological need. The release of PDGF from blood platelets in order to stimulate the division of skin cells is an example of such a normal signaling process. In contrast, some tumor cells produce growth factors that stimulate their own proliferation (Fig. 3.3). In such cases, abnormal growth-factor production leads to continual self-stimulation of cell division, and the cancer cells proliferate in the

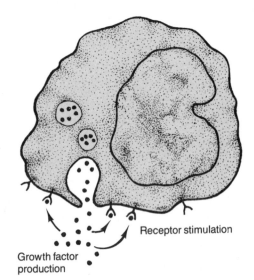

Figure 3.3

Growth-factor production by cancer cells. Some cancer cells produce growth factors to which they also respond, resulting in continual self-stimulation of cell division.

Receptor stimulation

Growth factor production

absence of growth factors from other, physiologically normal, sources. Some cancer cells, for example, produce PDGF, thus continuously driving their own uncontrolled proliferation.

Other cancer cells no longer require growth-factor stimulation due to malfunctions in other cell regulatory systems. In these cases, signals that would normally be initiated by a growth factor binding to the cell surface are instead aberrantly generated within the cell in the absence of growth-factor stimulation. For example, in some cancer cells growth-factor receptors function abnormally, signaling cell division even in the absence of stimulation by the appropriate growth factor (Fig. 3.4).

In addition to being controlled by growth factors that stimulate cell proliferation, normal cells are also regulated by signals that inhibit their growth. Such signals include contact with other cells, as well as hormones that inhibit rather than stimulate cell division. Frequently, cancer cells have lost the ability to respond to such growth inhibitory signals and therefore continue proliferating even in the presence of factors that would stop normal cells from dividing.

In summary, cancer cells become increasingly independent of the signals that either stimulate or inhibit normal cell growth. The net result of these alterations is the characteristic uncontrolled growth of cancer cells, which behave as autonomous individuals rather than as integrated components of the body.

THE INVASIVENESS AND METASTATIC POTENTIAL OF CANCER CELLS

Cancer cells are characterized not only by their uncontrolled growth and division, but also by their ability to invade surrounding tissues and metastasize throughout the body. As discussed in preceding chapters, this ability to spread from one site to another is responsible for most cancer deaths. Several abnormalities of cancer cells contribute to their lethal malignancy.

One striking difference between normal cells and cancer cells is illustrated by the phenomenon known to scientists as contact inhibition. Normal cells move freely until they make contact with another cell. Once contact occurs, normal cells cease further movement and adhere to each other, forming an orderly array in which each cell is aligned with its neighbor. The behavior of normal cells is thus regulated by interactions with their neighbors, leading to the orderly association of cells in tissues and organs.

The movement of cancer cells, in contrast, is not inhibited by contact with other cells. Instead, cancer cells continue moving on their own course, migrating over adjacent cells and growing in disorderly,

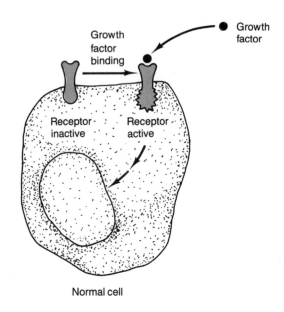

Normal cell

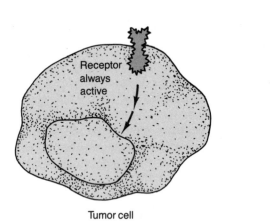

Tumor cell

Figure 3.4

Abnormal growth-factor receptors stimulate growth of cancer cells. Normal growth-factor receptors are activated by growth-factor binding; only then do they signal the cell to divide. However, growth-factor receptors of some cancer cells are active even in the absence of growth-factor binding, so they continuously signal cell proliferation.

multilayered patterns. Cancer cells thus fail to respond appropriately to interactions with their neighbors, contributing to their ability to invade surrounding normal tissues.

Another property of cancer cells playing an important role in invasion and metastasis is the production of enzymes that digest the proteins constituting barriers between the cancer cells and other tissues. Invasion and metastasis require that cancer cells pass through the walls of tissues and blood vessels, which are composed of a meshwork of proteins. The enzymes produced by cancer cells digest the proteins that make up this meshwork, thereby allowing the cancer cells to penetrate surrounding normal tissues and enter the circulation.

Both the growth and metastasis of cancer cells are also facilitated by the production of proteins that stimulate the growth of blood vessels in the vicinity of a tumor. This stimulation of surrounding blood vessels is critical to the growth of a tumor beyond the size of about 1 million cells. Once a tumor reaches this size, its further expansion requires the recruitment of new blood vessels to provide oxygen and nutrients to the growing mass of cancer cells. Such blood vessels are formed in response to growth factors produced by the cancer cells. These growth factors stimulate cells of the capillaries present in surrounding tissue, resulting in the growth of new capillaries into the tumor.

In addition to providing needed nutrients, the new blood vessels play a direct role in metastasis. In particular, the actively growing capillaries formed in response to a tumor are easily penetrated by the cancer cells. Thus, these new blood vessels provide a ready opportunity for tumor cells to enter the circulatory system and metastasize to distant body sites. The ability of cancer cells to induce formation of new blood vessels is therefore a critical determinant of both tumor growth and metastasis. Consequently, one new strategy being considered for cancer therapy is the use of drugs that inhibit this step in tumor development.

DEFECTIVE DIFFERENTIATION AND IMMORTALITY

Another important characteristic of cancer cells is that they generally fail to develop—differentiate—normally into specialized cell types. As discussed above, cell differentiation is the specialization of cells to perform particular tasks, for example, to function as nerve cells or muscle cells. The defective differentiation of cancer cells is closely related to their uncontrolled proliferation, since most fully differentiated cells either cease division or divide only slowly. Rather than carrying out their normal differentiation program, cancer cells are characteristically blocked at an early stage of the differentiation process, consistent with their continued growth and division.

The leukemias (cancers of blood cells) provide good examples of the relationship between defective differentiation and cancer (*Fig. 3.5*). There are several different kinds of blood cells, all of which are derived from the division of a common type of cell in the bone marrow. Descendants of these cells become committed to specific differentiation pathways. For example, some cells form red blood cells, whereas others form the various types of white blood cells. All of these cell types undergo several rounds of division as they differentiate, but once they become fully differentiated, cell division ceases. Leukemic cells, in contrast, fail to differentiate normally. Instead, they become arrested at an early stage of the differentiation process, at which they retain their capacity for proliferation and continue to divide. Interestingly, as will be discussed further in chapter 10, one type of leukemia can now be treated with a drug that induces differentiation of the leukemic cells, thereby blocking their continued proliferation.

For many types of cells, including blood cells, cell death is an integral part of their differentiation program. Some white blood cells, for example, live for only a few days, and continual division of precursor cells in the bone marrow is required to maintain populations of these cells at the appropriate levels. In such cases, the regulation of cell death is as critical to maintaining a constant cell population as is the regulation of cell division. Coincident with their failure to differentiate normally, cancer cells generally fail to die on schedule, instead continuing to proliferate indefinitely—a property referred to as cancer cell immortality. The progressive growth of cancer cells is thus a combined result of not only uncontrolled cell division but also the failure of cancer cells to undergo normal differentiation and programmed cell death.

GENETIC INSTABILITY AND TUMOR PROGRESSION

As discussed in chapter 2, the development of cancer is a multistep process; malignancy is the eventual result of a series of changes. Each of the steps in the process of tumor progression is thought to result from a mutation leading to increasingly abnormal cell behavior, such as more rapid growth or the enhanced ability to invade other tissues. It is therefore noteworthy that the genetic material of cancer cells is frequently less stable than normal. This genetic instability leads to a high frequency of mutations, which sometimes result in increased cell proliferation or other characteristics of malignancy. Cancer cells are thus prone to become more and more abnormal, leading to the increasingly rapid progression of malignant tumors.

The genetic instability of cancer cells is important not only in the development of cancer but also in its treatment. As will be discussed in

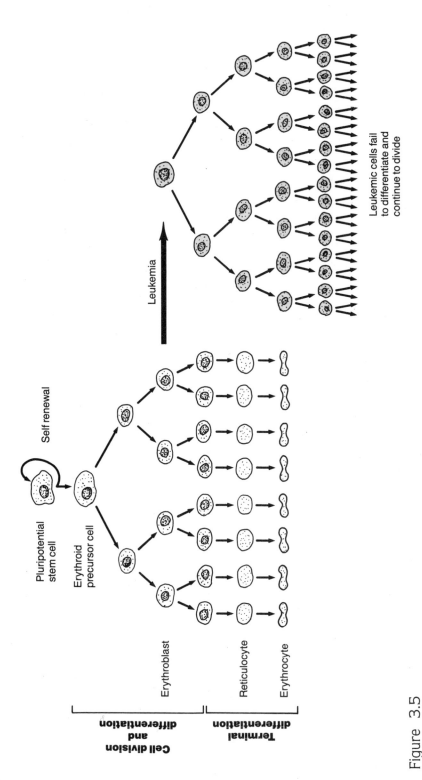

Figure 3.5

Defective differentiation in leukemia. Red blood cells (erythrocytes), like other blood cell types, are derived from a common cell (the pluripotential stem cell) in bone marrow. Normal erythrocyte precursor cells (erythroblasts) undergo cell division as they differentiate, but cell division ceases at the terminal stages of the differentiation process (reticulocytes and erythrocytes). In contrast, the differentiation of leukemic cells is blocked at an early stage, so they continue to divide.

detail in chapter 10, one of the problems commonly encountered in cancer chemotherapy is the development of drug resistance. In other words, the growth of many tumors is initially stopped by treatment with a drug, but the tumor then becomes resistant to the drug during the course of therapy. This results from the emergence of mutant, drug-resistant cells within the tumor cell population. In contrast to the initial, drug-sensitive tumor cells, which are killed by the chemotherapeutic drug administered, the growth of drug-resistant mutant cells is unaffected. Consequently, the drug-resistant cells continue to divide, gradually becoming the predominant cell type in the tumor. Once this occurs, the tumor no longer responds to the chemotherapeutic drug. Since drug-resistant cells arise as a result of mutations, the genetic instability of cancer cells is an important factor leading to their appearance. Consequently, the genetic instability of cancer cells poses a major problem in the successful treatment of cancer, as well as in its development.

SUMMARY

The growth and differentiation of normal cells is carefully regulated so that each cell functions in the best interests of the body as a whole. In order to achieve this regulation, cells are capable of sensing signals from their environment and responding appropriately. Such signals include contact with neighboring cells as well as a variety of hormones and growth factors. Most growth factors act by binding to the cell surface. A cell-surface receptor then generates signals that are transmitted to the nucleus, resulting in changes in the expression of genes that ultimately control cell division.

This careful regulation of cell behavior is lost in cancer cells. Rather than responding appropriately to the signals that control normal cells, cancer cells proliferate in an unregulated manner. In general, cancer cells are able to divide independently of the hormones and growth factors that control normal cell division, and are less stringently regulated by contact with neighboring cells and tissue components. The growth, invasion, and metastasis of cancer cells is further facilitated by their ability to dissolve the walls of tissues and blood vessels, and to recruit new blood vessels into the vicinity of a growing tumor. Cancer cells are also generally defective in differentiation and fail to undergo programmed cell death. Instead, their differentiation is blocked at early stages, compatible with continued cell division. Finally, cancer cells are characterized by genetic instability, which contributes to continuing tumor progression as well as the development of resistance to chemotherapeutic drugs.

PART II

Causes of Cancer

Chapter 4

Cancer and the Environment

The preceding chapters have described cancer as a family of diseases characterized by uncontrolled cell proliferation. What causes a normal cell to become cancerous? Since only limited success has been achieved in treating most cancers, the possibility of preventing cancer by identifying and eliminating the causative agents is obviously an important alternative.

As discussed earlier, the development of cancer is a multistep process that involves a series of mutations leading to the formation of tumor cells with increased proliferative capacity, invasiveness, and metastatic potential. Since many steps are required for the development of malignancy, it is overly simplistic to speak of single agents as the cause of any given cancer. It is much more likely that multiple factors contribute to cancer development, each acting to increase the likelihood of any step in the series of events that culminate in malignancy. A number of different factors, called risk factors, may therefore affect the likelihood that any given individual will develop cancer. Such risk factors include the genetic makeup of the individual as well as the environmental agents.

It is generally thought that the risk of developing many cancers is substantially affected by environmental agents, broadly defined as any external substance to which an individual is exposed. Environmental factors thus encompass all of the agents routinely encountered in the course of daily living, including substances present in food, air, and water. This chapter will consider chemicals, including dietary factors, and radiation as risk factors for human cancer. The role of viruses will be discussed in chapter 5, and genetic susceptibility to cancer in chapter 6. The mechanisms of action of some environmental agents will be further considered in chapter 7, and the development of strategies for cancer prevention, including dietary modification, will be the subject of chapter 8.

HOW CHEMICALS CAUSE CANCER

Agents that cause cancer (either chemicals or radiation) are called carcinogens. Such agents can act in two general ways to increase the likelihood that cancer will develop (Fig. 4.1). As discussed in chapters 2 and 3, tumors develop as a consequence of mutations that lead to the abnormal proliferation of cancer cells. Damage to a cell's genetic material (DNA) is thus a critical event in the development of cancer, and many carcinogens

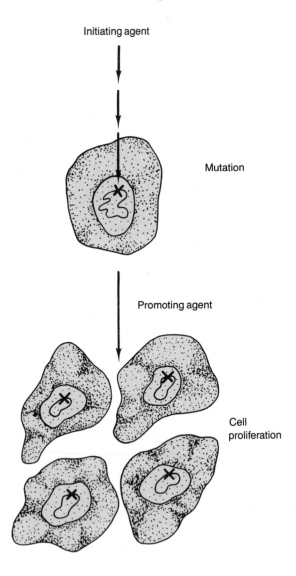

Figure 4.1

The action of carcinogens. Some carcinogens, called initiating agents, react with DNA to induce mutations, whereas others, called promoting agents, stimulate cell proliferation.

are agents that react with DNA to induce mutations. When such muta-tions alter the function of critical cell regulatory genes (discussed in chapter 7), the outcome can be abnormal cell growth, leading to cancer.

Other chemicals contribute to the development of cancer not by induc-ing mutations but by stimulating cell proliferation. The increased cell division resulting from exposure to these chemicals enhances the initial outgrowth of a population of tumor cells, thereby stimulating tumor development. Particularly important among these agents are hormones, especially estrogen. For example (as discussed further below), abnormal hormonal stimulation of cell proliferation by estrogen is a major factor in the development of endometrial cancer of the uterus.

In addition to agents that act to induce mutations or stimulate cell pro-liferation, some chemicals increase the risk of cancer by inhibiting nor-mal function of the immune system. As discussed in chapter 2, the immune system, the body's natural defense against a variety of infec-tions, also appears capable of acting against cancer cells, thereby pre-venting tumor growth. Consequently, chemicals or other agents that interfere with normal immune function impart an increased risk that cancer will develop.

Although many different agents can induce cancer in experimental animals in laboratory studies, a much more limited number appear to be important contributors to the development of most cancers in humans. This chapter will therefore focus on the major environmental sources of exposure to chemicals and radiation known to contribute to human can-cer risk.

THE IMPORTANCE OF ENVIRONMENTAL
FACTORS IN CANCER RISK

A principal argument linking cancer to environmental factors has come from comparisons of cancer incidence in different parts of the world. The important finding of such comparisons is that the frequency of spe-cific kinds of cancer varies markedly—often more than ten-fold—between different national populations. For example, the worldwide incidence of colon cancer is highest in the United States (annual rate of 34 per 100,000) and lowest in India (annual rate of 1.8 per 100,000)—a nineteen-fold difference.

In principle, such variation in cancer incidence could be due either to genetic differences between the national populations or to variation in environmental factors to which the inhabitants of different countries are exposed. In some cases, these alternative possibilities have been distin-guished by studies of migrant populations. For example, an informative comparison can be made between the incidence of some of the common cancers in the United States and Japan. Breast and colon cancers are among the most common cancers in the United States but rare in Japan. Conversely, stomach cancer, which is rare in the United States, is the most common cancer in Japan. Thus, the contribution of environmental versus genetic factors to these differences can be assessed by analysis of cancer incidence in the sizable populations of Japanese who have moved to Hawaii and California. In fact, within one to two generations, the incidence of cancers in these Japanese-Americans shifts from the Japanese to the American pattern. The characteristic patterns of cancer incidence in Japan compared to the United States therefore appear to be determined primarily by environmental factors rather than by genetic differences.

Similar changes in the pattern of cancer incidence are observed among other migratory populations, suggesting that the worldwide variations in cancer frequencies are primarily due to environmental differences. On this basis, it has been estimated that environmental factors are responsible for up to 80 percent of all cancers. At least in principle, then, many cancers could be prevented by identifying and eliminating the causative agents. The identification of environmental carcinogens has therefore received a great deal of emphasis in cancer research.

SMOKING AND CANCER

Cigarette smoking is unquestionably the major identified cause of human cancer, accounting for nearly one-third of all cancer deaths. Smoking is directly responsible for the vast majority (80–90%) of lung cancers. Since lung cancer is the most frequent lethal cancer in the United States, accounting for approximately 25 percent of all cancer deaths, it follows that a substantial fraction of total cancer mortality could be prevented by eliminating tobacco-induced lung cancer. As if this were not striking enough, smoking has also been implicated in the development of several other kinds of cancer, including cancer of the oral cavity, pharynx, larynx, esophagus, bladder, kidney, and pancreas. Combining the mortality from these cancers with that of lung cancer, it is estimated that smoking causes about 30 percent of all cancer deaths—clearly an impressive toll for a single environmental agent.

As noted in chapter 1, the incidence of lung cancer has increased more than ten-fold since 1930. This is closely correlated with the increased use of tobacco in the early part of this century, as illustrated in Fig. 4.2. A notable feature of this comparison is the lag time, about twenty years, between the increase in smoking and the resultant increase in lung cancer incidence. This lag time reflects the gradual, multistep development

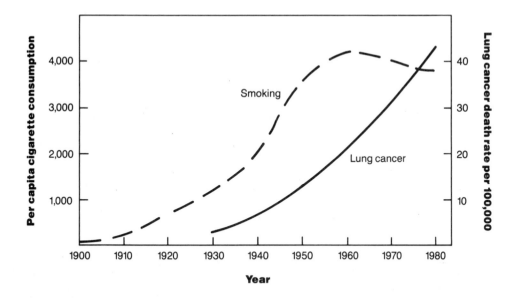

Figure 4.2

Cigarette smoking and lung cancer. Average annual per capita cigarette consumption and lung cancer death rates are shown for both sexes in the United States. (Data are from U.S. Dept. of Health and Human Services, *Reducing the health consequences of smoking: Twenty-five years of progress. A report of the Surgeon General, 1989.*)

of cancer, as discussed in chapter 2, and is characteristic of carcinogen-induced human cancers. Generally, it takes twenty to thirty years or more for a cancer to develop following exposure to a carcinogen.

The cause and effect relationship between cigarette smoking and lung cancer is further illustrated by considering differences between men and women with respect to both smoking habits and lung cancer incidence. Cigarette smoking by young men in the United States began to increase around 1910, whereas cigarette smoking did not become popular among women until around 1940. This thirty year difference is directly reflected in lung cancer incidence. Lung cancer in men began to increase about 1930, whereas lung cancer in women remained low until around 1960. In both men and women, increased incidence of lung cancer followed increased cigarette consumption with a characteristic twenty-year lag time.

The risk of developing lung cancer depends on both the extent and duration of smoking, as illustrated in Fig. 4.3. The mortality rate from lung cancer among heavy smokers (two or more packs a day) is about twenty times greater than for nonsmokers. The risk for moderate smokers

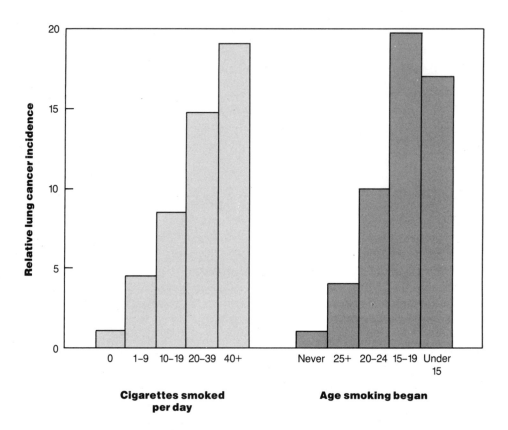

Figure 4.3

Relationship between lung cancer risk and the extent and duration of cigarette smoking. The lung cancer incidence for smokers is shown relative to that of nonsmokers. (Data are from the ACS twenty-five-state study, U.S. Dept. of Health and Human Services, *The health consequences of smoking: Cancer. A report of the Surgeon General,* 1982.)

(one-half to one pack per day) is about half that of heavy smokers. The effect of duration of smoking on lung cancer incidence is even more dramatic. For example, the risk for an individual who began smoking at age 15 is nearly five-fold greater than that of someone who began smoking after age 25. Thus, prolonged exposure is a major factor in tobacco-induced lung cancer, suggesting that cigarette smoke may contribute to several stages of tumor development.

Several other smoking variables also affect cancer incidence. The risk of lung cancer for smokers who inhale deeply is about twice that of smokers who inhale only slightly. Smoking filtered cigarettes with reduced tar and nicotine may also be associated with a lower cancer risk, but this does not produce a large difference. The risk of lung cancer for pipe or cigar smokers is less than that for cigarette smokers, although still greater than for nonsmokers. The effect of smoking pipes or cigars on the incidence of other cancers, however, is similar to that of smoking cigarettes. The use of smokeless tobacco (for example, snuff) also increases cancer incidence, particularly that of oral cancer. In addition, exposure to the smoke of others, called involuntary or passive smoking, may be associated with increased lung cancer risk, although the magnitude of this effect is much less than that of voluntary smoking.

Consistent with the role of prolonged exposure to cigarette smoke, the risk of lung cancer is substantially reduced by stopping smoking (Fig. 4.4). For an exsmoker, the risk of lung cancer remains about the

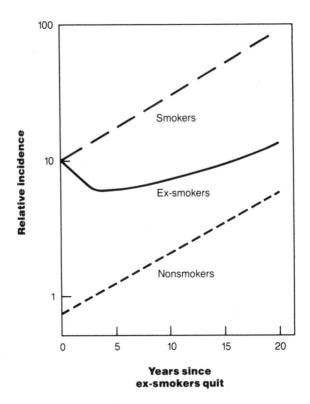

Figure 4.4

Lung cancer risk for exsmokers. The relative incidence of lung cancer among exsmokers, smokers, and nonsmokers is shown for twenty years after the exsmokers quit smoking. (From U.S. Dept. of Health, Education, and Welfare, *Smoking and health: A report of the Surgeon General*, 1979.)

same as it was at the time of quitting, rather than continuing to increase with age. After about twenty years, the lung cancer risk for an exsmoker becomes similar to that for a nonsmoker—approximately ten-fold lower than if smoking had continued.

The evidence implicating tobacco as a major cause of human cancer is abundantly supported by experimental studies in animals. Such studies have shown that tobacco smoke contains a variety of very potent carcinogenic chemicals, which can act to both induce mutations and stimulate cell proliferation. There is simply no question that smoking is the cause of a major proportion of human cancer mortality.

ALCOHOL

Excessive consumption of alcoholic beverages is clearly associated with an increased risk of some cancers, particularly those of the oral cavity, pharynx, larynx, and esophagus. In addition, excess alcohol consumption can result in cirrhosis, leading to an increased incidence of liver cancer, probably as a consequence of excess cell proliferation resulting from chronic tissue damage.

The effect of alcohol on the development of oral, pharyngeal, laryngeal, and esophageal cancers seems to be exerted largely in combination with that of smoking (Fig. 4.5). For example, the risk of oral and pharyngeal cancer is increased less than two-fold by either moderate smoking (1–2 packs per day) or moderate drinking (1–2 drinks per day) alone. In combination, however, moderate smoking and moderate drinking result in more than a four-fold increased risk of developing these cancers. Heavy smoking (more than 2 packs per day) or heavy drinking (more than 4 drinks per day) each increase the risk of oral and pharyngeal cancers six- to seven-fold, while heavy drinking and heavy smoking together result in an increased risk of nearly forty-fold.

The combination of alcohol and smoking thus exerts a greater effect than either alone, suggesting that each enhances the carcinogenic activity of the other. As will be noted in subsequent sections, many carcinogens behave in a similar cooperative, or synergistic, fashion. Consequently, the risk associated with combined exposure to multiple carcinogenic substances is frequently much greater than that associated with each substance by itself.

Alcohol is only weakly carcinogenic in experimental animals, acting mainly to potentiate the action of other carcinogens, so the mechanism by which excessive consumption of alcoholic beverages increases human cancer risk is not known. In addition to alcohol itself, it is possible that

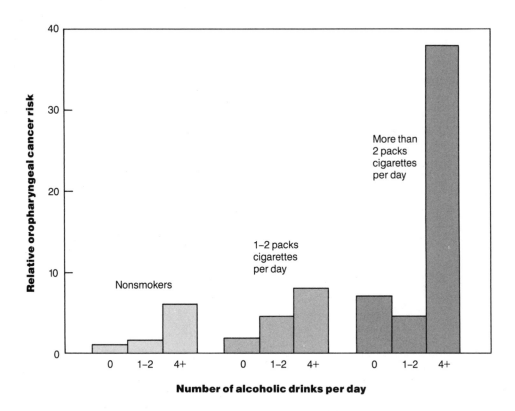

Figure 4.5

Combined effect of alcohol and smoking on oropharyngeal cancer. The risk of oropharyngeal cancer is shown relative to that of nonsmokers and nondrinkers. (From W. J. Blot et al., Smoking and drinking in relation to oral and pharyngeal cancer, *Cancer Res.* 48: 3282–3287, 1988.)

other ingredients of alcoholic beverages are carcinogenic. In any event, the association between consumption of alcoholic beverages and human cancer is well established. For example, the combination of alcohol and tobacco accounts for about 75 percent of all oral and pharyngeal cancers, which corresponds to over 6000 deaths per year in the United States. Since most heavy drinkers are also heavy smokers, it is difficult to determine the number of cancers that can be attributed to alcohol alone. Overall, however, it has been estimated that alcohol may be a contributory factor in up to 3 percent of United States cancer deaths.

RADIATION

Solar radiation, in the form of ultraviolet light, is the major cause of human skin cancer. As discussed in chapter 1, skin cancer is extremely common but seldom lethal. The incidence of the most common types of skin cancer—the nonmelanoma skin cancers—is approximately 600,000 cases per year in the United States. Almost all are thought to be induced by exposure to sunlight. For comparison, note that the incidence of lung cancer in the United States is approximately 160,000 cases per year, so solar radiation causes even more cancers than does smoking. Fortunately, however, the common nonmelanoma skin cancers metastasize very slowly and are consequently highly curable. This is reflected in the fact that these cancers result in only about 2500 deaths per year in the United States. In contrast, lung cancer is highly lethal, resulting in over 140,000 deaths annually in this country. Therefore, although nonmelanoma skin cancers caused by solar radiation are extremely frequent, they account for a comparatively small fraction of cancer mortality.

Exposure to excess sunlight is also associated with melanoma, which is a much more serious form of skin cancer since it rapidly spreads to other parts of the body. The annual incidence of melanoma in the United States is currently about 27,000 cases, resulting in about 6,000 deaths per year. But the incidence of melanoma is steadily increasing, both in the United States and throughout the rest of the world. Excessive exposure to sunlight thus appears to be a significant contributor to cancer mortality; it is associated with perhaps 1 to 2 percent of cancer deaths in the United States.

In addition to ultraviolet light, other forms of radiation can also cause cancer. In particular, the carcinogenic activity of higher energy forms of radiation (ionizing radiation), including x-rays and radiation produced by the decay of radioactive particles, is well established. The induction of cancer by these forms of radiation has been demonstrated not only in laboratory animals but also in humans exposed to excess radiation in a variety of unfortunate circumstances. For example, radiologists who used x-rays extensively in the early part of this century, before the danger was realized, suffered a three- to four-fold increased risk of leukemia. The carcinogenic effect of radiation produced by the decay of radioactive elements has likewise been demonstrated in several instances, including the increased rates of a number of cancers observed among the survivors of the World War II atomic bombings of Hiroshima and Nagasaki.

As with other carcinogens, the risk of developing cancer from exposure to ionizing radiation is related to the amount of radiation an individual receives. In assessing the carcinogenic potential of radiation exposure, it is important to recognize that different kinds of radiation vary both in their ability to penetrate tissue and in the amount of biological damage they cause. Radiation exposure is therefore usually considered in terms of the amount of radiation absorbed by tissue, corrected for the biological effectiveness of the particular form of radiation being considered.

About 80 percent of the ionizing radiation to which individuals in the United States are exposed is from natural sources, including cosmic rays and radioactive substances in the earth's crust. Medical sources, particularly diagnostic x-irradiation, account for most of the rest of radiation exposure for the general population. About 250 million x-ray exams are performed each year in the United States, so diagnostic x-irradiation is clearly a significant source of radiation exposure. However, since the carcinogenic potential of x-irradiation has been recognized, appropriate precautions have effectively reduced the exposure and risk associated with medical x-rays for both physician and patient. The average radiation dose in diagnostic exams is now quite low, and the risk associated with such exposure is correspondingly small, estimated to be as low as one induced cancer per 1 million x-ray examinations. According to this estimate, diagnostic x-irradiation would be responsible for approximately 250 cancers per year—less than 0.1 percent of total cancer mortality. This figure is imprecise, however, and may be in error by as much as several-fold. In any event, although reducing exposure to medical x-rays is one effective way to avoid radiation, the relatively small risk of diagnostic x-irradiation must be weighed against the benefits derived from this procedure.

As discussed in chapter 10, x-rays and other forms of radiation are frequently used for treatment of cancer. Such radiation therapy involves the use of much higher doses of radiation than diagnostic x-rays and is designed to kill the tumor cells. These higher doses carry a correspondingly higher probability of causing a second cancer to develop in the patient. However, it is again necessary to weigh risk against benefit. It is generally felt to be more urgent to treat the cancer that a patient already has than it is to worry about the possibility that a new cancer might later develop.

A major source of radiation exposure for the general population is radon gas in the home, which accounts for three to four times more radiation than is received from medical x-rays. Radon is a natural source of radiation, formed as a decay product of uranium, which can seep into homes from underground. Radioactive decay products can then attach to aerosol particles, be inhaled, and become lodged in the lung. The carcinogenic effect of radon appears to combine with that of cigarette smoking, so the increased risk of lung cancer resulting from radon exposure is primarily observed among smokers. It has been estimated that radiation resulting from exposure to radon in United States homes may contribute to up to 10,000 lung cancer deaths per year—about 2 percent of total cancer mortality. Levels of indoor radon, and thus the associated risk, vary widely (over 1000-fold) in homes throughout the country. Many homes have much higher than average levels of radon, which is associated with substantially increased risks of lung cancer. Identification and modification of such homes to reduce indoor radon levels could be expected to significantly reduce cancer risk.

DIET

Variations in diet are an obvious possibility in accounting for the differences in cancer incidence between national populations. Many potential carcinogens are found in foods, whereas other dietary components may help to prevent the development of cancer. A great deal of public and media attention has been focused on the role of diet in cancer. And indeed, it has been estimated that up to 30 percent of total cancer deaths in the United States are related to dietary factors. A number of food components have been suggested to either increase or decrease cancer risk

Table 4.1
DIETARY FACTORS AND CANCER RISK

Dietary Component	Effect on Cancer Risk
High fat	Increased risk of colon and possibly breast cancer
High calorie	Obesity resulting in increased risk of endometrial and possibly breast cancer
Cured, smoked, and pickled foods	Increased risk of stomach cancer
Aflatoxin	Increased risk of liver cancer
Vitamin A or β-carotene	Decreased risk of lung and other epithelial cancers
Vitamin C	Decreased risk of stomach cancer
Vitamin E and selenium	Deficiencies associated with increased cancer risk
Fiber	Decreased risk of colon cancer
Cruciferous vegetables	Decreased cancer risk

(Table 4.1). However, in contrast to the clear identification of tobacco, alcohol, and radiation as carcinogens, attempts to define specific dietary agents that affect cancer incidence have yielded controversial and contradictory results. Consequently, the role of potential dietary carcinogens as causes of human cancer has not yet been conclusively established.

Dietary Fat

Diets that are high in calories and fat have been repeatedly linked to increased cancer incidence. The association is strongest for dietary fat, which may contribute to development of breast and colon cancers. One indication of this relationship comes from comparing fat consumption with cancer incidence in different national populations. For example, there is a strong correlation between dietary fat intake and breast cancer frequency in different countries. The drawback of such correlations, however, is that there are many other differences besides fat intake between the countries under study. For example, most countries with high rates of breast cancer also have higher levels of economic development. Consequently, there is also a good correlation between gross national product and breast cancer incidence, although this is not taken to indicate that economic development causes cancer. The question that must therefore be asked concerning such comparisons is whether dietary fat is the real cause of high breast cancer rates. Alternatively, dietary fat might only be incidentally associated with some other, unknown factor that represents the true cause of increased cancer frequencies.

The possibility that dietary fat is directly associated with increased cancer incidence has been supported by studies with experimental animals. For example, breast cancer incidence is substantially higher in mice that are fed a high-fat diet. On the other hand, a number of studies have failed to correlate fat intake with tumor incidence in humans within the same national population. For example, one large study involved almost 90,000 United States women. During a four-year period, 601 cases of breast cancer were diagnosed within this group. Analysis of the dietary practices of these women failed to reveal any significant difference in fat intake between those women who developed breast cancer and those who did not. Although other studies have indicated that high fat intake may be associated with about a 1.5-fold increase in breast cancer risk, the potential association between high fat diets and breast cancer incidence remains equivocal.

The association between high fat diets and colon cancer risk, however, has been more reproducibly demonstrated. For example, analysis of the same group of United States women referred to above indicated that colon cancer was nearly twice as frequent among those whose diet contained approximately 44 percent of calories as fat than among those whose diet contained only 30 percent calories as fat.

Although statistically significant in at least some studies, the associations between dietary fat and breast or colon cancer risk are clearly much less than the twenty-fold increased risk of lung cancer that results from heavy cigarette smoking. On the other hand, since breast and colon cancer claim the lives of over 100,000 Americans per year, even a modest reduction in the risk of developing these cancers would result in a significant decrease in total cancer mortality. Unfortunately, there remain substantial inconsistencies between different studies. Although there is generally thought to be a correlation between high fat diets and increased risk of some cancers, particularly colon cancer, the extent to which high fat intake contributes to human cancer incidence remains unclear.

Obesity

Cancer of the uterine endometrium is associated with excess body weight, reflecting a high calorie diet. For example, the risk of endometrial cancer has been estimated in different studies to be two- to five-fold higher for women weighing more than 165 pounds than for women weighing less than 125 pounds. The basis for this association may be hormone production by fat cells. Endometrial cancer is associated with increased levels of estrogens—hormones produced by the ovaries—which act to stimulate proliferation of endometrial cells of the uterus. But fat cells also produce estrogen, and significantly contribute to estrogen levels in postmenopausal women. Consequently, production of this hormone by fat cells is thought to provide a link between obesity (defined as body weight 40% in excess of normal) and endometrial cancer. Although estrogen also stimulates the proliferation of epithelial cells of the breast, excess body weight is associated with only a modest increase (less than 1.5-fold) in breast cancer risk, suggesting the importance of other factors as critical determinants of breast cancer development.

Dietary Factors that Reduce Cancer Risk

In contrast to dietary fat and high calorie intake, other dietary components, including dietary fiber, certain vitamins, selenium, and other compounds present in some vegetables have been suggested to reduce cancer risk. In general, it appears that diets rich in fresh fruits and vegetables are associated with decreased cancer incidence. Such diets are high in fiber, carotenoids (a source of vitamin A), and vitamin C, as well as being low in fat and calories. Studies evaluating the putative roles of individual dietary factors, however, have generally been inconclusive.

Dietary Fiber

The possibility that dietary fiber protects against colon cancer has been investigated since the 1970s. A number of studies have suggested that the risk of colon cancer is reduced about two-fold by consumption of foods that are rich in dietary fiber, including vegetables, fruits, and grains. Other studies, however, have failed to detect any protective effect of dietary fiber. Moreover, it is unclear whether the anticancer effects that have been associated with high fiber diets are in fact due to fiber or to other vegetable components. Studies in experimental animals have been similarly inconclusive: some experiments indicate that fiber exerts a protective effect, but others do not. Overall, it appears likely that diets rich in fiber are associated with a reduced risk of colon cancer, but this protective effect cannot unequivocally be attributed to fiber per se.

Vitamin A

Vitamin A and related compounds have been shown to block the development of a variety of cancers in experimental animals. Diets that are rich in β-carotene, which is metabolized to form vitamin A, are associated with a decreased incidence of several cancers, including those of the lung, esophagus, stomach, bladder, and breast. The evidence is strongest for lung cancer, and several studies have indicated that diets deficient in green and yellow vegetables (which are rich in β-carotene) are associated with up to a two-fold increase in lung cancer risk. It is not clear, however, whether these protective effects are due to β-carotene itself, to vitamin A, or to other vegetable components. It should be noted, however, that, as discussed in chapter 8, compounds related to vitamin A have been found in trial chemoprevention studies to reduce the frequency of secondary head and neck cancers (e.g., cancers of the oral cavity, pharynx, and larynx) among a population of patients who had been treated for one such cancer and were at high risk of developing a second. It thus appears that compounds related to vitamin A can act to inhibit the development of cancer in both experimental animals and humans. Importantly, however, the doses of vitamin A that have been found effective in inhibiting the development of cancer are much higher than those available in normal dietary sources. This is particularly problematic, since the high doses of vitamin A used in both animal and human chemoprevention studies produce a number of toxic side effects.

Vitamin C

Possible anticancer effects of vitamin C have received a great deal of public attention, but there is only limited support for such claims. Some, but not all, studies have found a modest protective effect (less than two-fold) of citrus fruit against stomach cancer, but it is unclear whether this is due to vitamin C or to other food components, possibly including vitamin A. Although vitamin C has been found to protect against the development of cancer in some laboratory studies, the same effects have not been observed in other experiments.

Vitamin E and Selenium

Other vitamins have not been shown to reduce cancer incidence, although deficiencies of vitamin E, combined with low levels of selenium, may increase the risk of a variety of cancers. Selenium is a trace element derived from soil, and it has been observed that geographic areas with low selenium levels are associated with increased cancer incidence. Some studies have found that low blood levels of selenium in individual patients are also correlated with about a two-fold increase in cancer risk, although these findings are not yet extensive enough to be conclusive. A possible anticancer role for selenium is further supported by laboratory experiments, which suggest that high levels of dietary selenium protect against cancer development. At high doses, however, selenium is toxic, so caution must be employed in extrapolating such potential protective effects to human use.

Cruciferous Vegetables

Several other vegetable components, in addition to fiber and vitamins, may also protect against cancer. In particular, cruciferous vegetables, including broccoli, Brussels sprouts, cabbage, cauliflower, collards, kale, mustard greens, rutabagas, turnips, and turnip greens, contain several compounds that inhibit the action of carcinogens in experimental animal studies. These compounds may contribute to the protection against cancer conferred by vegetable-rich diets.

Cured, Smoked, and Pickled Foods

In addition to considerations of general dietary balance, a number of food additives have been considered potential carcinogens. An increased incidence of stomach cancer has been associated with consumption of cured, smoked, and pickled foods, which contain large amounts of salt, nitrates, and nitrites. The specific carcinogenic component associated with these foods is not known, but it is noteworthy that nitrites can be readily converted to a class of chemicals, nitrosamines, which are known to be potent carcinogens in animal studies. Vitamin C inhibits the formation of these compounds, however, perhaps accounting for its suggested protective effect against stomach cancer.

Aflatoxin and Liver Cancer

Contaminants present in food can also be carcinogenic. A good example is provided by aflatoxin, a compound produced by some molds, which can grow in improperly stored supplies of peanuts and grains. Aflatoxin is an extremely potent carcinogen in animals, and contaminated food supplies have been associated with liver cancer in humans. More specifically, studies in Africa and Asia have shown that high rates of liver cancer in different geographic areas are directly correlated with exposure to aflatoxin, to the extent that the risk of liver cancer is about five-fold higher in areas with high levels of aflatoxin contamination in foods. In the United States, however, the levels of aflatoxin contamination are minimal and are not likely to contribute significantly to cancer incidence.

Other Potential Carcinogens in Food

A number of additional dietary components, both natural and synthetic, can act as carcinogens, at least in animal tests. However, the role of these compounds in human cancer is not established. A good case in point is the artificial sweetener saccharin. Animal tests have clearly shown that high doses of saccharin cause bladder cancer in rats. However, the amount of saccharin required to induce these cancers is 100- to 1000-fold greater than the amounts consumed by humans, and studies of possible correlations between saccharin use and human bladder cancer have been negative. It thus appears that, although saccharin is a potential dietary carcinogen, its normal use does not in fact confer increased cancer risk. Other potential carcinogens present in food include food colorings, pesticides, carcinogens produced during cooking (particularly during broiling meat and fish), and a variety of natural carcinogens present in food plants. There is presently no evidence that any of these substances makes a significant contribution to cancer incidence in the United States.

General Dietary Recommendations

Although dietary factors are believed to contribute to a sizable proportion of cancers, attempts to identify specific components which either increase or decrease human cancer incidence have largely been inconclusive. It is also unclear whether children are more susceptible to some potential dietary carcinogens than adults, perhaps because of their lower body weight or the high rate of cell proliferation in growing tissues. At present, the clearest dietary risk factors are high-fat diets (for colon cancer), obesity (for endometrial cancer), and smoked, cured, and pickled foods (for stomach cancer).

General dietary recommendations designed to reduce cancer risk have been made by a number of expert panels, such as the American Cancer Society. Such recommendations (discussed further in chapter 8) include reducing fat intake, eating fruits, vegetables, and high-fiber foods, and minimizing consumption of smoked, pickled, and cured foods. Such advice constitutes good general health practice and therefore represents a reasonable and prudent course of action despite the fact that the actual effects of such dietary recommendations on cancer incidence are not definitive.

MEDICINES THAT CAUSE CANCER

The increased risk of cancer associated with exposure to radiation from medical x-rays was discussed earlier in this chapter. Similarly, some medications have been found to increase the risk of cancer as a side effect of their actions on the cells of the patient receiving treatment. In total, it is estimated that such medications may account for up to 1 percent of the total cancer incidence in the United States. Some of these cancer-causing drugs have been eliminated from current practice, although other potentially carcinogenic medicines remain in use because their therapeutic effects outweigh their possible dangers.

Hormones, in particular estrogens, have been a significant cause of some human cancers. An especially notable instance was the administration of diethylstilbestrol (DES), a synthetic estrogen, to pregnant women in the 1940s and '50s. In the early 1970s, it was discovered that the daughters of women who had received diethylstilbestrol during pregnancy had an increased incidence of vaginal and cervical cancers. Fetal exposure to this hormone led to the development of cancer ten to twenty years later.

In current practice, administration of diethylstilbestrol to pregnant women has, of course, been eliminated. However, estrogens are frequently still used to alleviate symptoms of menopause and to prevent osteoporosis (bone thinning). Postmenopausal estrogen replacement therapy, particularly long-term treatment with high doses of estrogen alone, significantly increases the risk of endometrial cancer, and therefore needs to be carefully considered from the standpoint of relative risk to benefit. Fortunately, this risk is substantially reduced by treatment with lower doses of estrogen in combination with progesterone, which

counteracts the stimulatory effect of estrogen on endometrial cell proliferation. Postmenopausal estrogen administration may also increase the
risk of breast cancer, but this is a more modest effect (less than 1.5-fold)
and has not been conclusively established.

Estrogens are also the chief ingredient of birth control pills. Substantially increased rates of endometrial cancer were associated with an
early form of the pills, which contained only estrogen in relatively high
doses. These pills were removed from the market in the 1970s. The birth
control pills currently available contain lower doses of estrogen in combination with progesterone, and the use of these combination pills is not
associated with increased endometrial cancer risk. In fact, the incidence of
endometrial cancer is actually decreased among users of these combination oral contraceptives, presumably due to the inhibition of endometrial
cell proliferation by progesterone. Most studies have found no association
between breast cancer incidence and use of oral contraceptives, although
some studies have suggested a modest increase in risk associated with
long-term use of birth control pills prior to first pregnancy.

Anticancer drugs are themselves frequently carcinogenic. As will be
discussed in chapter 10, many of these drugs damage the genetic material of the cell and, consequently, sometimes cause mutations that can
convert a normal cell into a cancerous one. As noted above, however,
regarding the use of radiation in cancer therapy, the benefits of anticancer drugs generally far outweigh the possibility that they will induce
development of a second cancer.

Drugs that suppress function of the immune system are used in organ
transplant procedures to prevent rejection of the donor tissue. Studies of
transplant patients have indicated that they suffer increased risk of some
types of cancer, particularly lymphomas and Kaposi's sarcoma, a generally rare form of cancer that is also seen in AIDS patients. These cancers
thus appear to develop much more readily in the absence of normal
immune function.

OCCUPATIONAL CARCINOGENS

Some of the clearest examples of environmental carcinogens are occupational carcinogens—agents to which groups of workers are exposed in
high doses. The first observation of an occupational carcinogen was made
in 1775 by the British physician Percival Pott, who noted a high incidence
of scrotal cancer in young men who had been employed as chimney
sweeps when they were children. Pott attributed these cancers, correctly,
to the effect of soot that became lodged in the folds of the scrotum. Eventually, the identification of this occupational carcinogen led to preventive

measures; the incidence of scrotal cancer declined when chimney sweeps began to wear protective clothing and to bathe regularly.

Since then, occupational carcinogens have been relatively easy to identify because, as in the case of scrotal cancer, a high incidence of a particular kind of cancer becomes apparent in a specific group of workers. Consequently, studies of occupational carcinogens have identified more causes of human cancer than any other approach (Table 4.2). Once occupational carcinogens are recognized, appropriate actions can be taken to limit exposure by affected workers. Unfortunately, as discussed in preceding sections, there is generally a long lag time between exposure to a carcinogen and the development of a resulting cancer. Thus, a significant number of workers still suffer increased risks of cancer due to earlier exposure to occupational carcinogens that have since been recognized and controlled. In total, occupational exposure to carcinogens may account for up to 5 percent of cancer mortality.

A good example of an occupational carcinogen is provided by asbestos, which is still widely used in the construction industry. The association between asbestos and lung cancer was first suggested in the 1930s and became clear by the 1950s, when it was recognized that factory workers who were heavily exposed to asbestos suffered as much as tenfold increased rates of lung cancer. Further studies have shown that the effect of asbestos on lung cancer, like that of radon and many other carcinogens, appears to combine with the effect of smoking. The first United States regulation limiting asbestos exposure in the workplace was put in place in the late 1960s, and the regulations have since been made increasingly stringent. However, since the lag time between exposure to asbestos and development of lung cancer can be thirty years or more, the effects of occupational exposure to high, unregulated levels of asbestos are still being felt.

ENVIRONMENTAL POLLUTION

A large number of chemicals have been introduced into the environment as industrial pollutants. Many of these chemicals can induce cancer in experimental animals and must, therefore, be considered potential human carcinogens. In addition, most of the chemicals known to act as occupational carcinogens are also released into the environment as pollutants and might thereby lead to increased cancer risk for the general population. Fortunately, however, these potential carcinogens are generally present at very low levels, and it does not seem likely that they are substantial contributors to total cancer incidence.

One line of argument suggesting that industrial pollution has not had a substantial impact derives from the analysis of cancer rates over the

Table 4.2
OCCUPATIONAL CARCINOGENS

Carcinogen	Occupational Exposure	Cancer Risk
4-Aminobiphenyl	Chemical and dye workers	Bladder
Arsenic	Mining, pesticide workers	Lung, skin, liver
Asbestos	Construction workers	Lung
Auramine	Dye workers	Bladder
Benzene	Leather, petroleum, rubber, and chemical workers	Leukemia
Benzidene	Chemical, dye, and rubber workers	Bladder
Bis(chloromethyl) ether	Chemical workers	Lung
Chromium	Metal workers, electroplaters	Lung
Isopropyl alcohol	Manufacturing by strong-acid process	Nasal
Leather dust	Boot and shoe manufacturing and repair	Nasal, bladder
Mustard gas	Mustard gas workers	Lung, larynx, nasal
Naphthylamine	Chemical, dye, and rubber workers	Bladder
Nickel dust	Nickel refining	Nasal, lung
Radon	Underground mining	Lung
Soots, tars, and oils	Coal, gas, and petroleum workers	Lung, skin, bladder
Vinyl chloride	Rubber workers, polyvinyl chloride manufacturing	Liver
Wood dusts	Furniture manufacturing	Nasal

last fifty years. As noted in chapter 1, the incidence of most cancers has remained relatively constant since 1930. Lung cancer is an exception, having increased dramatically, but this is directly attributable to cigarette smoking. The absence of increasing rates for other major cancers suggests that industrial waste products introduced into the environment over this time period have not notably increased cancer incidence. However, given the usual lag time of twenty years or more between carcinogen exposure and cancer development, the effects, if any, of recently introduced pollutants may not yet be apparent.

Comparisons of cancer incidence in urban and rural areas similarly suggest that industrial pollution is not a major cancer risk factor. The overall incidence of lung cancer is higher in industrialized cities than in the country, initially suggesting the possibility that industrial pollution contributes to lung cancer risk. However, these differences appear instead to be primarily a result of an earlier increase in cigarette smoking among city dwellers. When populations with similar smoking habits are compared, the rates of lung cancer in urban and rural environments are not significantly different. A good example is provided by comparing lung cancer incidence in Finland and Britain. Despite a much greater degree of industrial pollution in Britain, the rates of lung cancer in the two countries are similar, consistent with similar levels of cigarette consumption by the two national populations. It therefore appears that, in spite of the many potential carcinogens introduced into the air by industrial processes, air pollution in cities has not made a substantial contribution to overall cancer rates.

Consideration of the quantities of potential carcinogens released into the environment also suggests that pollution is not likely to be a major cause of cancer. An illustrative comparison is provided by noting that the amount of potentially carcinogenic burnt material inhaled per day by breathing Los Angeles smog is equivalent to smoking only one-tenth of a cigarette. As discussed earlier in this chapter, the effect of smoking on lung cancer is strongly dose-dependent, and this level of smoking would not constitute a significant risk. Similar comparisons can be made between the amounts of industrial pollutants present in the general environment and those to which workers are exposed. For example, the level of asbestos generally present in city air is more than 1000 times less than that currently permitted for occupational exposure.

Pollution has also introduced a number of carcinogens into drinking water, including known occupational carcinogens such as benzene and vinyl chloride. However, the amounts of these chemicals in drinking water are, again, very small compared to those in the workplace, and consequently do not seem likely to represent any significant carcinogenic risk.

All of these considerations lead to the conclusion that industrial pollution is not a major cause of human cancer. On the other hand, the number of potential carcinogens introduced into the environment by pollution is large, and entire populations are exposed to these agents throughout their lifetimes. Moreover, the carcinogenic results of pollution are clearly evident in other animal species, particularly fish, which are exposed to higher amounts of industrial waste than are humans. For example, flounder in contaminated sites of Boston Harbor have a high incidence of liver cancer, apparently resulting from exposure to chemical pollutants. It, therefore, clearly seems prudent to control the release of carcinogens into the environment by reasonable regulations. The appropriate level of concern about environmental pollution in relation to cancer, however, is a matter of some controversy, which will be further discussed in chapter 8.

SUMMARY

Comparisons of cancer incidence in different countries suggest that up to 80 percent of human cancers may be attributable to environmental risk factors. The major identified cause of human cancer is tobacco use, primarily cigarette smoking, which accounts for approximately 30 percent of total cancer mortality in the United States. Other identified risk factors for human cancer include radiation, excessive alcohol consumption, carcinogenic medicines, and occupational carcinogens, each of which accounts for only a few percent of total cancer deaths. Taken together, these known carcinogens account for about 35 to 40 percent of United States cancer mortality, which corresponds to about half of the total fraction of cancers (80%) estimated to be associated with environmental factors. A substantial portion of the remaining half may be related to diet, but specific dietary risk factors for most cancers have not been conclusively identified.

Chapter 5

Viruses, Cancer, and AIDS

The environmental risk factors for human cancer include viruses, in addition to chemicals and radiation. Viruses are the simplest and smallest forms of life. They are not cells and cannot grow and divide on their own. Instead, they multiply by infecting cells of a host organism and taking over the cellular machinery to produce more virus particles. Therefore, viruses can be considered parasites that reproduce inside cells by subverting normal cellular functions. In many cases, viruses kill the cells in which they replicate. Sometimes, however, cells are not killed by virus infection but are instead altered to become cancer cells. Most viruses, including those that cause the common cold, polio, and influenza, do not cause cancer. Nevertheless, a number of viruses are known to induce cancer in experimental animals. Moreover, several kinds of viruses are associated with specific types of human cancers (Table 5.1). The role of these viruses in human cancer will be the subject of this chapter.

Table 5.1
VIRUSES ASSOCIATED WITH HUMAN CANCERS

Virus	Type of Cancer
Hepatitis B virus (HBV)	Liver cancer
Human papillomaviruses (HPV)	Cervical and other anogenital cancers, rare skin cancers
Epstein-Barr virus (EBV)	Burkitt's and other B-cell lymphomas, nasopharyngeal carcinoma
Human T-cell leukemia virus (HTLV-1)	Adult T-cell leukemia
Human immunodeficiency virus (HIV)	Lymphomas, Kaposi's sarcoma, anogenital cancers

HEPATITIS B VIRUS AND LIVER CANCER

Hepatitis B virus is the major risk factor for liver cancer and is responsible for a substantial fraction of human cancer worldwide. Hepatitis B virus specifically infects liver cells and can cause acute liver damage. In 5 to 10 percent of cases, infection with hepatitis B virus is not resolved, and a persistent, chronic—usually lifelong—infection of the liver can develop. Such infection imparts a high risk of liver cancer to chronic hepatitis B virus carriers.

Although rare in the United States and Europe, liver cancer is extremely common in other parts of the world, particularly in parts of Asia and Africa. For example, the annual incidence of liver cancer in the United States is less than 4 per 100,000 people, whereas its incidence in China, Korea, and parts of Africa is as high as 150 per 100,000—a difference of more than thirty-fold. Throughout the world, it has been estimated that there are 250,000 to 1 million cases of liver cancer annually. Liver cancer is thus one of the most frequent human cancers overall, accounting for 5 to 15 percent of worldwide cancer incidence.

The strong correlation between the frequency of hepatitis B virus infection and the incidence of liver cancer was established through comparative studies in different countries (Fig. 5.1). For example, about 10 percent of adults in the United States have been infected with hepatitis B virus, and less than 1 percent are chronic carriers. In contrast, virtually 100 percent of adults in China have been infected, and 10 to 15 percent are virus carriers. These differences in the frequency of chronic infection clearly correlate with the much higher incidence of liver cancer in China.

Comparisons of the frequency of liver cancer in chronically infected versus uninfected individuals in the same national populations further substantiate the role of hepatitis B virus inferred from cross-national studies. For example, a study of over 20,000 Chinese showed that liver cancer was more than 200-fold more frequent among chronic hepatitis B virus carriers. In addition, hepatitis B virus is regularly found in cancerous liver cells, consistent with the idea that infection with this virus contributes directly to changing a normal liver cell into a cancer cell.

The role of hepatitis B virus in human liver cancer is also supported by studies in experimental animals. A member of the hepatitis B virus family has been shown to cause liver cancer in woodchucks, and it has been demonstrated that introduction of human hepatitis B virus into mice can also lead to liver cancer in this species.

Thus, a variety of different types of studies convincingly demonstrate the role of hepatitis B virus as a causative agent of liver cancer. In areas

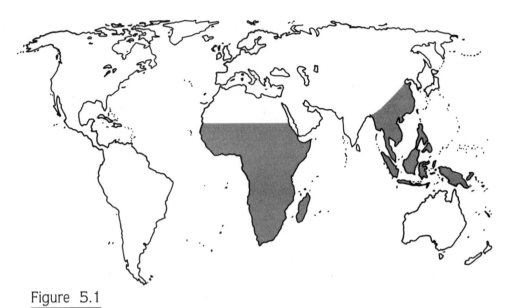

Figure 5.1

Worldwide distribution of hepatitis B virus and liver cancer. Areas of the world with a high frequency of hepatitis B virus infection also have a high incidence of liver cancer.

with high frequencies of hepatitis B virus infection, chronic carriers usually become infected early in life, although cancer does not develop until around 40 years of age. As in the case of chemicals and radiation, there is a lag time of several decades between initial infection with hepatitis B virus and the eventual development of cancer. Other factors, such as alcohol and aflatoxin (discussed in chapter 4), may also contribute to liver cancer risk. But the role of hepatitis B virus as a major risk factor is clear. Worldwide, more than 250 million people are chronic hepatitis B virus carriers and, consequently, suffer more than a hundredfold increased risk of developing liver cancer.

PAPILLOMAVIRUSES AND CERVICAL CANCER

The papillomaviruses are a common group of viruses that cause both benign and malignant tumors in several species of animals. The first of these viruses to be isolated caused benign skin tumors—papillomas—in rabbits. In humans, approximately sixty different types of papillomaviruses, which infect cells of several tissues, have been identified (Table 5.2). Some of these viruses cause only benign tumors such as com-

Table 5.2
EXAMPLES OF HUMAN PAPILLOMAVIRUSES

Virus Type	Associated Tumor
HPV-1 and 4	Plantar warts
HPV-2, 7, 27, and 29	Common warts
HPV-3, 10, 26, and 28	Flat warts
HPV-5 and 8	Skin cancer in patients with epidermodysplasia verruciformis
HPV-6 and 11	Genital warts
HPV-16, 18, and 33	Anogenital cancers

mon skin warts, whereas others are important causative agents of malignant tumors, particularly cancer of the cervix and other anogenital sites.

Many different types of human papillomaviruses can infect skin cells and cause warts (Table 5.2). Generally, skin warts are benign growths that do not become malignant. However, in patients with a rare skin disease, known as epidermodysplasia verruciformis, malignant tumors frequently develop from the warts induced by some types of human papillomaviruses. Thus, in this unusual circumstance, infection with some human papillomaviruses can lead to skin cancer development.

The critical link between papillomaviruses and common human cancers, however, was the identification of other types of human papillomaviruses as causative agents of cervical cancer. Epidemiological data had suggested for many years that cervical cancer was a sexually transmitted disease. For example, cervical cancer is extremely rare among nuns and most frequent among women who have had multiple sexual partners. In addition, the risk of cervical cancer is increased for women married to men whose former wives have had the disease. Such correlations strongly indicated that cervical cancer is caused by a sexually transmitted infectious agent such as a virus.

The causative agent resisted identification, however, until 1983, when a distinct papillomavirus, human papillomavirus type 16, or HPV-16, was first isolated from a cervical cancer specimen. Subsequent studies also detected specific types of human papillomaviruses in several anogenital cancers, including those of the vulva, penis, and anal region as well as the cervix. HPV-16 is the most frequent type of virus found, being present in approximately 50 percent of these tumors. Another 20 percent of these cancers contain HPV-18, 10 percent contain HPV-33, and 10 percent contain other human papillomavirus types. Thus, all told, about 90 percent of anogenital cancers are associated with papillomavirus infection. Interestingly, genital infection with different types of human papillomaviruses has quite distinct pathological consequences. For example, HPV-6 and HPV-11 cause genital warts which almost always remain benign, whereas infection with HPV-16 or HPV-18 appears to confer a high risk of progression to malignancy.

The association of human papillomaviruses with genital cancers is supported by a variety of experimental studies that clearly demonstrate the cancer-causing potential of these viruses. It thus appears that some types of human papillomaviruses are causative agents of lethal malignancies, the most frequent of which is cervical cancer. But, as in the case of hepatitis B virus and other carcinogens, there is a lag time of several decades between primary papillomavirus infection and cancer development.

As noted in chapter 1, the mortality from cervical cancer is declining in the United States; it currently accounts for only about 1 percent of total cancer deaths. This decline is due, in large part, to the early diagnosis and treatment made possible by the Pap smear. Worldwide, however, cervical cancer is much more common, accounting for approximately 460,000 cases per year, or about 7 percent of total cancer incidence.

EPSTEIN-BARR VIRUS, THE IMMUNE SYSTEM, AND LYMPHOMAS

Epstein-Barr virus was the first virus recognized as a cause of human cancer. It is associated with Burkitt's lymphoma in regions of Africa, with nasopharyngeal cancer in parts of China, and with lymphomas in immunosuppressed individuals, including patients suffering from AIDS. Although most of the cancers caused by Epstein-Barr virus are confined to highly restricted geographic areas, infection with the virus is common throughout the world. In most areas, including the United States, Epstein-Barr virus infection of normal individuals does not lead to cancer. The fact that this virus is a major cancer risk factor in specific geographic regions, therefore, indicates that other factors must also contribute to tumor development.

Burkitt's lymphoma is a childhood cancer which, although rare throughout most of the world, is the most frequent cancer in African children, occurring with an annual incidence of up to 10 cases per 100,000 children in some areas (Fig. 5.2). In these high-incidence areas, infection with Epstein-Barr virus is clearly associated with lymphoma development. First, virtually all Burkitt's lymphomas in African children contain Epstein-Barr virus. In addition, an extensive study of over 40,000 Ugandan children has demonstrated a close correlation between infection with Epstein-Barr virus and subsequent development of Burkitt's

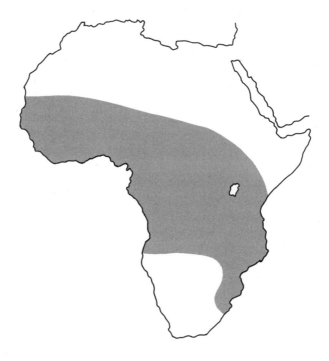

Figure   5.2

Regions of Africa with a high incidence of Burkitt's lymphoma caused by Epstein-Barr virus.

lymphoma, after a lag time of several years. These epidemiological associations are further supported by experimental studies, which demonstrate the ability of Epstein-Barr virus to cause cancer in a variety of laboratory tests.

Although Burkitt's lymphoma is common only in regions of Africa, over 90 percent of people throughout the world have been infected with Epstein-Barr virus. Outside of Africa, however, infection with this virus generally causes no disease or causes mononucleosis, not cancer. In mononucleosis, the Epstein-Barr virus infects and stimulates proliferation of the same kind of cells, B lymphocytes, that give rise to Burkitt's lymphoma. Proliferation of these cells in mononucleosis, however, is limited, and they do not become malignant. Thus, Epstein-Barr virus infection is clearly not sufficient by itself to cause Burkitt's lymphoma, and some other factor must contribute to the high incidence of the disease in regions of Africa.

One possibility is that malaria, which is widespread in those same regions of Africa, contributes to development of this cancer, by interfering with normal function of the immune system. This possibility is consistent with the increased frequency of lymphomas in immunodeficient patients in non-African countries. Individuals who lack a normally functioning immune system, either because of genetic abnormalities (see chapter 6), medical treatments (e.g., suppression of immune function to prevent rejection of organ transplants), or infection (e.g., AIDS), have a high risk of developing lymphomas that are associated with Epstein-Barr virus. It is thus possible that Epstein-Barr virus infection of a normal individual results in only mononucleosis, where the proliferation of infected lymphocytes is limited by normal immune function. In the absence of a normal immune system, however, infection with the same virus may lead to continual lymphocyte proliferation, culminating in malignancy.

Another kind of cancer, nasopharyngeal cancer, is also caused by Epstein-Barr virus. This cancer is common in China, where it occurs with an annual incidence of about 10 per 100,000—a frequency about 100 times higher than in the United States. Epstein-Barr virus is found in nearly all nasopharyngeal cancer specimens, and development of the disease in China appears to be closely associated with Epstein-Barr virus infection. As in the case of Burkitt's lymphoma in Africa, however, other factors must be invoked to explain why infection with this virus results in a high incidence of nasopharyngeal cancer specifically in the Chinese population.

HUMAN T-CELL LEUKEMIA VIRUSES

The human T-cell leukemia viruses are members of a large family of viruses, called retroviruses, that cause a variety of cancers in several different animal species. The ability of retroviruses to cause cancer was first discovered in experimental animals (chickens) in 1908, and members of this virus family have been studied for many years because of their ability to induce cancer in laboratory experiments. Only within the last decade, however, have retroviruses that cause human cancer been identified.

Human T-cell leukemia virus type 1, or HTLV-1, has been identified as the causative agent of adult T-cell leukemia, a disease that is rare in the United States and Europe but frequent in parts of Japan, the Caribbean, and Africa. The virus was initially isolated from patients with this disease, and epidemiological studies have provided strong evidence for its causal role. They have shown that HTLV-1 is prevalent in those geographic areas that have a high incidence of adult T-cell leukemia, and have established that infection with the virus is closely correlated with development of the disease. For example, adult T-cell leukemia occurs

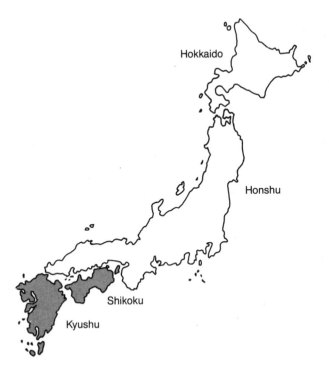

Figure 5.3

Islands of Japan with a high frequency of HTLV-1 infection and a high incidence of adult T-cell leukemia.

with high incidence in the two southwestern islands of Japan, Shikoku and Kyushu, but not in the rest of the country (Fig. 5.3). Virtually all individuals with the disease are infected with HTLV-1, as are approximately 20 percent of the healthy individuals on these two islands. In contrast, infection with HTLV-1 is rare in the rest of Japan—only 1 to 2 percent of healthy individuals are infected—as it is in the United States and Europe. There is thus a clear relationship between infection with HTLV-1 and development of adult T-cell leukemia, which occurs with a characteristic lag time of many years after initial infection with the virus. In addition to this strong epidemiological evidence, HTLV-1 is reproducibly found in tumor cells of adult T-cell leukemias and has readily demonstrable cancer-causing potential in laboratory studies.

A related virus, HTLV-2, may also be associated with human T-cell leukemia, but the evidence for its role as a cause of human cancer is much less clear. HTLV-2 has been isolated from two unusual cases of a particular kind of leukemia, called hairy T-cell leukemia. Like HTLV-1, HTLV-2 has been shown capable of causing cancer in laboratory experiments. In contrast to HTLV-1, however, HTLV-2 has not been epidemiologically associated with the occurrence of leukemia. Its role in human cancer is therefore uncertain.

AIDS AND CANCER

Acquired immune deficiency syndrome—AIDS—is caused by another human retrovirus, human immunodeficiency virus, or HIV. AIDS is not itself a cancer, nor does HIV infection appear to cause cancer directly by converting a normal cell into a cancerous one. However, AIDS patients suffer an extremely high incidence of certain types of cancer. These cancers seem to develop as a consequence of immunodeficiency and, therefore, represent a secondary effect of HIV infection.

HIV, like HTLV, infects a type of lymphocyte (the T4 cell), which is an important component of the functional immune system. In contrast to HTLV, however, HIV does not cause these cells to proliferate and become cancerous. Instead, HIV kills the cells in which it replicates, eventually resulting in depletion of the population of T4 lymphocytes in an infected individual. The result of depletion of these lymphocytes is immune deficiency. In the absence of a normally functioning immune system, AIDS patients are sensitive to infection by a variety of agents to which a healthy individual would be resistant. Moreover, AIDS victims suffer a high frequency of the same types of cancers that are also seen in other immunosuppressed individuals, for example, patients who have undergone organ transplants (see chapter 4).

The most frequent type of cancer encountered in AIDS patients is Kaposi's sarcoma, a tumor that is extremely rare among the general population. Kaposi's sarcoma develops in approximately 15 percent of AIDS patients, a frequency about 20,000 times higher than in normal individuals. Notably, the incidence of Kaposi's sarcoma in AIDS patients is also significantly higher, by about a hundred-fold, than in other immunosuppressed individuals. The particularly high incidence of this neoplasm in AIDS patients may be due both to the effects of immunosuppression and to the fact that HIV-infected lymphocytes appear to produce factors that specifically stimulate the growth of Kaposi's sarcoma cells.

Lymphomas are the second most common cancer associated with HIV, occurring in up to 10 percent of AIDS patients. In this case, the incidence of lymphoma in AIDS patients is similar to that in other immunosuppressed individuals. The majority of lymphomas in AIDS patients are caused by infection with Epstein-Barr virus, which, as discussed earlier in this chapter, leads to lymphoma development in the absence of normal immune function.

Anogenital cancers associated with human papillomavirus infection also occur frequently in patients with AIDS.

A high percentage of HIV-infected individuals thus develop cancer, particularly those types associated with infection by other viruses. In contrast to the other viruses discussed in this chapter, however, the tumors in AIDS patients are not induced by direct action of HIV in the cancer cell. Rather, they develop as a secondary consequence of immunodeficiency resulting from HIV infection.

SUMMARY

Four kinds of viruses act directly to cause human cancers. Two of these, hepatitis B virus and the papillomaviruses, cause cancers that are common worldwide. In particular, hepatitis B virus–induced liver cancer and papillomavirus-induced cervical cancer may account for 10 to 20 percent of overall cancer incidence. Cancers induced by Epstein-Barr virus and human T-cell leukemia virus (HTLV) are not common worldwide, but occur with high frequency in some geographic areas. In addition to these viruses, human immunodeficiency virus (HIV) indirectly causes a high frequency of Kaposi's sarcoma and lymphomas, which develop as a result of immunodeficiency in AIDS patients. A significant fraction of human cancers are thus caused by viruses. Worldwide, virus-induced cancers may account for up to one-fourth of the 80 percent of total cancers that can be attributed to environmental factors.

Chapter 6

Heredity and Cancer

The environmental agents—chemicals, radiation, and viruses—discussed in preceding chapters constitute major risk factors for many cancers. In most cases, the action of these agents leads to the development of cancer in otherwise normal individuals. Moreover, the vast majority of patients with cancer have not inherited the disease and do not pass it on to their children. Therefore, cancer, in general, is not considered a hereditary disease.

In spite of this generalization, there are a number of instances in which an individual's susceptibility to cancer is affected by heredity. These include, first, rare forms of cancer that are inherited directly. And several very rare genetic diseases, such as inherited immunodeficiencies, are also associated with striking predispositions to the development of cancer. In addition, less well characterized hereditary factors appear to affect susceptibility to many of the common cancers, including those of the breast, lung, and colon. An individual's risk of developing cancer may therefore be determined by genetic susceptibility as well as exposure to environmental carcinogens.

INHERITED CANCERS

Although directly inherited cancers constitute only a small percentage of total cancer incidence, there are rare hereditary forms of many different kinds of cancer (Table 6.1). In these cases, a strong predisposition to cancer is transmitted directly from parent to child, and development of cancer is inherited like any other genetic trait such as hair or eye color. Most of these inherited predispositions lead to the development of only one or a few specific types of cancer, not to all cancers in general. The mode of inheritance of these cancers suggests that susceptibility is determined by single genes that are transmitted in a genetically dominant fashion (Fig. 6.1). Thus, one-half of the children of an affected parent will inherit the cancer-susceptibility gene from that parent. Since cancer susceptibility is dominant, the children who have inherited this gene will almost always

Table 6.1
REPRESENTATIVE EXAMPLES OF INHERITED CANCERS

Genetic Disease	Types of Cancer
Beckwith-Wiedemann syndrome	Wilms' tumor, hepatoblastoma, rhabdomyosarcoma, adrenal tumors
Dysplastic nevus syndrome	Melanoma
Familial adenomatous polyposis	Colon cancer
Li-Fraumeni cancer family syndrome	Sarcomas, breast cancer, brain tumors, leukemia, adrenocortical tumors
Lynch cancer family syndrome	Breast and ovarian cancer
Multiple endocrine neoplasia-1	Pituitary, parathyroid, adrenal, and pancreatic tumors
Multiple endocrine neoplasia-2a	Pheochromocytoma, medullary thyroid carcinoma
Multiple endocrine neoplasia-2b	Pheochromocytoma, medullary thyroid carcinoma, mucosal neuroma
Neuroblastoma	Neuroblastoma
Neurofibromatosis Type 1 (von Recklinghausen's disease)	Neurofibrosarcoma, malignant Schwannoma
Neurofibromatosis Type 2	Acoustic neuroma, meningioma
Nevoid basal cell carcinoma	Basal cell skin cancer
Retinoblastoma	Retinoblastoma, osteosarcoma
Von Hippel-Lindau syndrome	Retinal and cerebellar angioma, kidney cancer
Warthin cancer family syndrome	Colon and endometrial cancer
Wilms' tumor (WAGR syndrome)	Wilms' tumor

develop cancer, even in the presence of a normal gene copy from the other parent. Such inherited cancers generally occur early in life, and affected individuals frequently develop multiple independent tumors.

Many of the inherited cancers are rare diseases of childhood. A good example is provided by retinoblastoma, an eye tumor that usually develops in children by the age of 3. Retinoblastoma is a tumor of embryonic retinal cells (*retino*=retinal, *blast*=embryonic cell, and *oma*=tumor). Provided that the disease is detected early, retinoblastoma can be successfully treated by surgery and radiotherapy, so most affected children now survive to have families. This has allowed inheritance of the disease to be

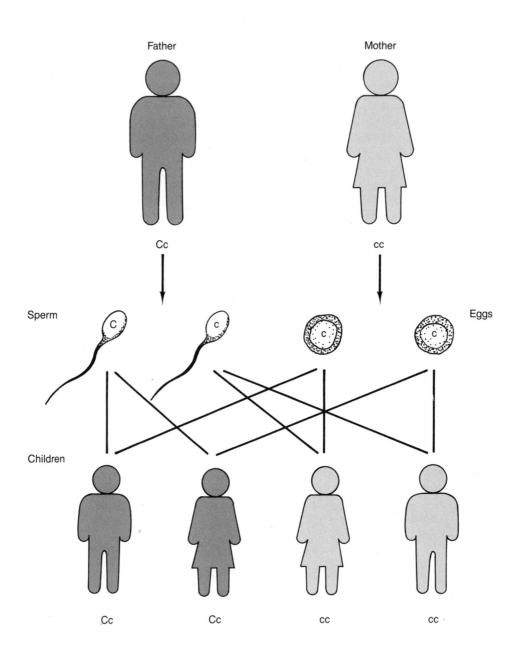

Figure 6.1

Inheritance of a cancer susceptibility gene. The gene for cancer susceptibility is designated C and its normal equivalent is designated c. In this example, one parent (the father) has one copy of C and one copy of c. Since C is dominant, he develops cancer. The mother is normal and has two copies of c. The father transmits the C gene to one-half of his children, resulting in cancer development.

studied by following the family history and offspring of retinoblastoma patients. Such studies have shown that retinoblastoma can occur in two forms: either as an inherited disease (Fig. 6.2) or in a sporadic, noninherited manner. Individuals with the inherited form of the disease transmit retinoblastoma to approximately one-half of their offspring. In contrast, sporadic retinoblastoma occurs without prior family history and is not transmitted to the patients' children. As is typical of the hereditary cancers, most children with inherited retinoblastoma develop multiple tumors in both eyes, whereas children with the sporadic form of the disease develop only a single tumor in one eye. In addition, children who have inherited the disease usually develop tumors at a younger age than do children with the sporadic form. Retinoblastoma is an infrequent disease, affecting about 1 in 20,000 children, with the inherited form accounting for about 40 percent of the total incidence.

Other childhood cancers for which hereditary forms are known, such as Wilms' tumor, a kidney cancer, also occur infrequently, affecting about 1 in 10,000 children. As in the case of retinoblastoma, patients with inherited Wilms' tumor usually develop multiple tumors in both kidneys. In contrast to retinoblastoma, however, less than 10 percent of Wilms' tumors (and other childhood cancers) are hereditary. Inherited cancers thus constitute a small fraction of total childhood cancer incidence.

Hereditary cancers are not limited, however, to the rare cancers of childhood. There are also inherited forms of many common adult cancers, including colon and breast carcinomas (Table 6.1). In these cases, the inherited forms account for no more than a few percent of total disease incidence.

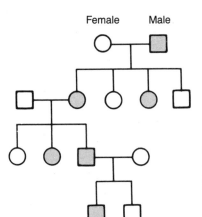

Figure 6.2

A family pedigree illustrating the inheritance of retinoblastoma. Affected individuals are indicated by filled symbols. In inherited retinoblastoma, the retinoblastoma susceptibility gene is transmitted to approximately one-half of offspring.

Colon cancer is a good example of a common cancer with both inherited and sporadic forms. About 1 in 20 Americans are affected by colon cancer, which occurs nearly 1000 times more frequently than the childhood cancers discussed above. The majority of colon cancers occur sporadically, but two inherited forms of the disease have been identified. The most frequently recognized is known as familial adenomatous polyposis (*adenoma* = benign epithelial tumor, and *polyp* = benign tumor projecting from an epithelial surface). This disease, like retinoblastoma, is inherited as a single dominant genetic trait. During the first twenty years of life, affected individuals develop hundreds of colon adenomas, or polyps. The likelihood that one or more of these multiple benign adenomas will progress to malignancy is extremely high, so that most affected individuals (more than 75%) develop colon cancer by age 40 if the disease is not treated. The colons of these patients are, therefore, usually removed before cancer has a chance to develop. The frequency of familial adenomatous polyposis is about 1 in 10,000, so this inherited form accounts for less than 0.5 percent of total colon cancer incidence. The second inherited form, hereditary nonpolyposis colon cancer, in which affected individuals develop colon cancer without the large number of polyps characteristic of familial adenomatous polyposis, is similarly infrequent. Thus, in spite of the existence of at least two inherited forms, over 95 percent of colon cancer appears to represent noninherited, sporadic disease.

Rare hereditary forms of most of the other common cancers, including leukemias and lymphomas, sarcomas, melanoma, brain tumors, and carcinomas of a variety of sites, are similarly transmitted as dominant genetic traits. Usually, a propensity to develop only one or a few kinds of cancer is inherited, but some hereditary predispositions lead to the development of multiple tumor types. An example of such multiple-tumor inheritance is the Li-Fraumeni cancer family syndrome, which refers to dominant inheritance of several types of tumors, primarily sarcomas and breast cancers, but also leukemias, brain tumors, adrenocortical tumors, and others (Fig. 6.3). Other cancer family syndromes include inherited predispositions to development of both breast and ovarian cancers (Lynch cancer family syndrome) and to both nonpolyposis colon and endometrial cancers (Lynch II or Warthin cancer family syndrome).

A wide variety of both childhood and adult cancers can thus be inherited. In each case, these inherited cancers are transmitted as single genes that impart a very high risk of tumor development. All of these hereditary forms of cancer are quite rare, however, so directly inherited cancers constitute only a small fraction of the total disease incidence.

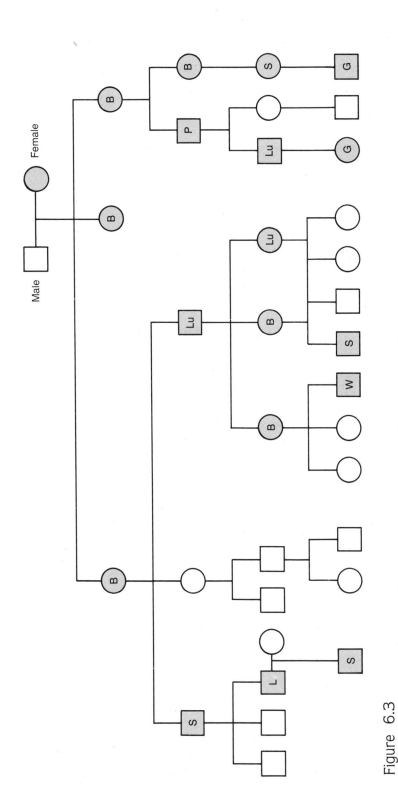

Figure 6.3

A pedigree of a family with Li-Fraumeni cancer family syndrome. Individuals with cancer are depicted by filled symbols. A blank symbol is cancer of unknown origin. B represents breast cancer; G, glioblastoma; L, leukemia; Lu, lung cancer; P, pancreatic cancer; S, sarcoma; and W, Wilms' tumor. (From F.P. Li and J.F. Fraumeni, Prospective study of a family cancer syndrome, *J. Amer. Med. Assoc.* 247:2692–2694, 1982).

Table 6.2
INHERITED PREDISPOSITIONS TO CANCER ASSOCIATED WITH
GENETIC INSTABILITY

Genetic Disease	Types of Cancer
Ataxia telangiectasia	Leukemias and lymphomas
Bloom's syndrome	Leukemias and lymphomas
Fanconi's anemia	Leukemias and squamous cell carcinomas
Xeroderma pigmentosum	Skin cancers

GENETIC DISEASES THAT PREDISPOSE TO CANCER

The hereditary cancers discussed above represent diseases in which the inherited genetic defect exerts a direct effect on the behavior of the cells that become cancerous. For example, as will be discussed further in chapter 7, the mutant gene whose inheritance leads to retinoblastoma directly affects proliferation of the retinal cells from which the tumor will develop. In contrast, other genetic diseases confer an indirect predisposition to increased cancer incidence. The primary disorders in these diseases affect either the stability of the cellular genetic material or the function of the immune system. A high frequency of tumor development is a secondary consequence of such defects in affected individuals. The diseases of this group also differ from the inherited cancers in their mode of genetic transmission. They are transmitted as recessive rather than dominant traits, so that the development of disease requires inheritance of two abnormal gene copies, one from each parent.

Xeroderma pigmentosum is a good example of a disease in which defective maintenance of the genetic material confers increased cancer susceptibility; in this case, to skin cancer (Table 6.2). Individuals with this disease suffer from several skin (*derma*) disorders, particularly extreme dryness (*xerosis*) and areas of nonuniform pigmentation (*pigmentosum*). The disease is extremely rare, with an incidence of only about 1 in 250,000. The basic defect in xeroderma pigmentosum is an inability to repair the genetic damage caused by ultraviolet light, which, as discussed in chapter 4, is the major environmental risk factor for skin cancer. Because of its inability to repair such damage, the skin of xeroderma pigmentosum patients is much more sensitive to solar radiation than that of normal individuals. As a result, individuals with this disease characteristically develop multiple skin tumors with high frequency. Other diseases of this general type, in which abnormalities in genetic maintenance lead to increased cancer incidence, include ataxia telangiectasia, Bloom's

Table 6.3
INHERITED IMMUNODEFICIENCY SYNDROMES

Genetic Disease	Types of Cancer
Ataxia telangiectasia	Leukemias and lymphomas
Common variable immunodeficiency	Lymphomas and stomach cancers
Severe combined immunodeficiency	Leukemias and lymphomas
Wiskott-Aldrich syndrome	Leukemias and lymphomas
X-linked agammaglobulinemia	Leukemias and lymphomas
X-linked lymphoproliferative syndrome	Lymphomas

syndrome, and Fanconi's anemia. The central feature of these diseases is that genetic damage occurs with an abnormally high frequency in affected individuals. Since the conversion of a normal cell to a cancer cell results from mutations in the genes regulating cell growth, the increased frequency of genetic damage leads to a high likelihood that cancer will develop.

The increased incidence of certain cancers resulting from a lack of normal immune function due either to immunosuppressive drugs or to AIDS was discussed in chapters 4 and 5. In addition to these immunodeficiencies, which are acquired, there are a number of diseases in which immunodeficiency is inherited (Table 6.3). Patients with inherited immunodeficiencies, like those with acquired immunodeficiencies, suffer an increased risk of developing cancer. The inherited immunodeficiency diseases include ataxia telangiectasia, so the increased cancer incidence seen in these patients may be due to both genetic instability and abnormal immune function.

Lymphomas, in particular, occur about one hundred times more frequently in immunosuppressed individuals. As discussed in chapter 5, some lymphomas are associated with Epstein-Barr virus infection. In normal individuals, the immune system effectively limits the proliferation of Epstein-Barr virus–infected cells, preventing lymphoma development. However, in immunodeficient individuals, Epstein-Barr virus infection leads to unlimited lymphocyte proliferation, eventually resulting in malignancy.

FAMILIAL SUSCEPTIBILITY TO CANCER

Both types of disorders discussed above—directly inherited cancers and genetic diseases that predispose to cancer development—are transmitted as single genes with well-defined patterns of inheritance. Inheritance of these genes results, either directly or indirectly, in a very high risk of cancer in affected individuals. In addition to these clearly inherited predispositions to cancer, other genetic determinants appear to exert weaker, but still significant, effects on cancer susceptibility. These inherited susceptibilities constitute important familial risk factors for some of the common cancers of adults.

Melanoma is a good example of a cancer for which there are clear-cut hereditary differences in susceptibility. The incidence of melanoma is about ten times higher among whites than among blacks. This difference probably reflects the greater degree of pigmentation of black skin, which provides substantial protection against the damage caused by solar ultraviolet radiation. An individual's risk of developing melanoma is thus determined by the combination of genetic susceptibility—skin pigmentation—and exposure to an environmental agent—sunlight. Genetic factors may also contribute to some of the other variations in cancer incidence among ethnic groups, such as the high incidence of Epstein-Barr virus–induced nasopharyngeal carcinoma among the Chinese (see chapter 5). As discussed in chapter 4, however, studies of migrant populations clearly indicate that most of the worldwide variation in cancer incidence is due to environmental rather than hereditary differences in national populations.

In addition to heritable racial differences in the incidence of certain kinds of cancer, there also appear to be familial risk factors for a number of common types. As discussed above, only rare cases of these cancers are directly inherited by transmission of single genes. There are, however, less well understood genetic determinants that affect susceptibility to the sporadic forms of several frequently occurring cancers, including those of the breast, lung, and colon. In these cases, the risk of developing cancer is generally increased two- to three-fold for individuals with first degree relatives (parents or siblings) who have had the disease. This increased familial risk is much less than that associated with the directly inherited forms of cancer. For example, the risk of developing colon cancer is increased more than 1000-fold by inheritance of familial adenomatous polyposis. The familial risk factors for common cancers thus appear to represent relatively small differences in cancer susceptibility. On the other hand, they represent a significant determinant of cancer risk for a much larger number of individuals than those affected by the rare cancers that are directly inherited.

Neither the genetic basis nor the mode of inheritance of these familial risk factors has yet been identified. Some risk factors in this category may represent inherited differences in an individual's sensitivity to carcinogens. For example, recent studies suggest that genetic differences in the ability to metabolize some of the chemicals in cigarette smoke may affect the risk of lung cancer by five- to ten-fold. Moreover, it is estimated that such inherited susceptibility may contribute to about 20 percent of all lung cancer cases. Genes that confer increased susceptibility to breast and colon cancers have also been estimated to be inherited by 10 to 20 percent of the population, and such inherited susceptibilities may play a role in the development of a substantial fraction, perhaps most, of these common adult tumors.

SUMMARY

Although the vast majority of cancers are not directly inherited, there are a number of ways in which susceptibility to cancer can be genetically transmitted. Rare, inherited forms of many childhood and adult cancers are transmitted as single genes that directly confer a high likelihood—virtually 100 percent—of development of particular tumors. Other rare hereditary diseases lead indirectly to the development of cancer, by affecting either the stability of cellular genetic material or the function of the immune system. Both of these types of inherited cancer susceptibilities are extremely rare and account for only a small fraction of total cancer incidence. In addition, however, heredity appears to govern some familial differences in susceptibility to the more frequently occurring cancers. Compared to the rare inherited cancers, such familial factors impart smaller increases in risk, but they may contribute to a significant fraction of common adult cancers.

Chapter 7

Genetic Changes in Cancer Cells

As discussed in preceding chapters, cancer is characterized by the uncontrolled growth of cells that fail to respond appropriately to the signals that regulate normal cell behavior. Such abnormal growth is the consequence of mutations, resulting in the aberrant function of critical cell regulatory genes. In rare cases (discussed in chapter 6), mutations that result in the development of cancer are genetically transmitted from parent to child. However, this is not usually the case. Most mutations leading to the development of cancer are not inherited, but occur in individual body cells during someone's lifetime. These mutations affect only the cells that eventually give rise to a tumor—they are not present in the sperm or eggs and are not transmitted to offspring. Some such mutations occur as a result of errors that take place during normal cell division. Others are induced by exposure to environmental agents, including chemicals, radiation, and some viruses.

As discussed in chapter 3, the behavior of normal cells is controlled by particular genes that regulate cell growth and differentiation in concert with the needs of the body as a whole. The mutations leading to the development of cancer alter the function of these critical regulatory genes, resulting in the uncontrolled proliferation and progressive spread characteristic of cancer cells. The identification of such genes has represented an area of major progress in cancer research over the last decade.

Scientists now recognize that there are two distinct classes of such genes, called oncogenes and tumor suppressor genes, and are beginning to understand their roles in both normal cell growth and the development of malignancy. Since these studies are providing a fundamental explanation of what goes wrong in cancer cells, they may form the basis of new approaches to cancer prevention and treatment. Indeed, as will be discussed in later chapters, our increasing knowledge of oncogenes and tumor suppressor genes is already being applied to the diagnosis and treatment of some types of cancer.

ONCOGENES

As discussed in chapter 3, normal cells are controlled by the action of genes which either stimulate or inhibit cell division. Oncogenes are formed as a result of mutations that increase the expression or activity of those genes that stimulate cell proliferation. Normally, the activity of these genes is regulated by appropriate signals from outside the cell so that they trigger cells to divide only as required to perform needed body tasks, for example, healing a cut. These genes can, however, be converted to oncogenes if they suffer mutations that result in unregulated activity. As a result of such mutations, oncogenes drive uncontrolled cell proliferation, thereby contributing to the development of cancer.

A good example of the activity of an oncogene is provided by the gene encoding platelet-derived growth factor (PDGF), which was introduced in chapter 3 as a protein that signals skin cells to divide. Normally, PDGF is released from blood platelets when blood clots. It then binds to a receptor on the surface of skin cells, triggering cell division. Thus, the normal action of PDGF is to signal skin cells to divide in order to repair damage resulting from a cut or wound. However, mutations sometimes convert the gene for PDGF to an oncogene. These mutations result in abnormal gene expression, so that a skin cell itself begins to produce PDGF (Fig. 7.1). This is decidedly abnormal, since PDGF is normally produced by blood platelets, not skin cells, and the result is uncontrolled cell growth. Since the skin cell also responds to PDGF, it has begun to produce a growth factor that drives its own proliferation. In this situation, therefore, the gene for PDGF acts as an oncogene. Its abnormal expression results in continual stimulation of cell proliferation, eventually leading to cancer.

As also discussed in chapter 3, growth factors like PDGF act by binding to specific receptors on the surface of responsive cells. Growth-factor binding activates the receptors, which then transmit signals through the cell to the nucleus, resulting in changes in the expression of other genes, which eventually lead to cell division. Genes encoding proteins that act at all levels of such regulatory pathways, not just growth factors themselves, can suffer mutations converting them to oncogenes. For example, genes encoding growth-factor receptors can be converted to oncogenes through mutations which result in their abnormal activity (Fig. 7.2). In such cases, the receptors encoded by the oncogenes are active even in the absence of growth-factor binding. Consequently, the cell is continually stimulated to divide, even without the growth factor normally required to signal cell division.

Thus, oncogenes can act at many different levels to drive inappropriate cell proliferation. Since the regulation of cell behavior is complex,

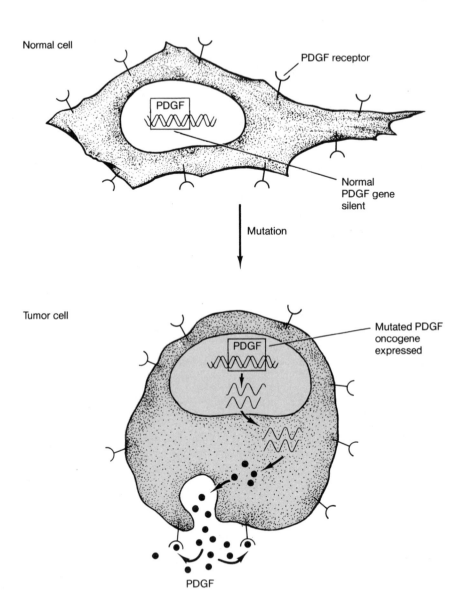

Figure 7.1

Action of PDGF as an oncogene. Normal skin cells express a receptor for PDGF but do not express the gene for PDGF itself. However, mutations in the PDGF gene can result in its abnormal expression. When this occurs, the mutated cell then produces the growth factor, to which it also responds, resulting in abnormal stimulation of cell proliferation.

many different oncogenes—over seventy—have been identified to date. Some function as growth factors, some as growth-factor receptors, and some at other levels of the pathways that signal cell division. At least twenty different oncogenes are regularly involved in human cancers, although some are more common than others (Table 7.1). The most common oncogenes in human cancers are called the *ras* genes. These oncogenes are involved in 15 to 20 percent of all cancers in the United States, including about 25 percent of lung cancers, 50 percent of colon cancers, 90 percent of pancreatic cancers, and 25 percent of acute leukemias. Other types of cancer, including breast cancers and many varieties of leukemias and lymphomas, frequently involve other oncogenes. Mutations resulting in the inappropriate expression or activity of a variety of different genes thus serve to drive abnormal growth and division of many types of cells, contributing to cancer development thereby. Such mutations can be induced by radiation or chemical carcinogens. In addition, many of the viruses which cause human cancer (discussed in chapter 5) act by introducing their own oncogenes into infected cells. The abnormal proliferation of cells stimulated by oncogenes is thus a common feature of cancers induced by a variety of different agents.

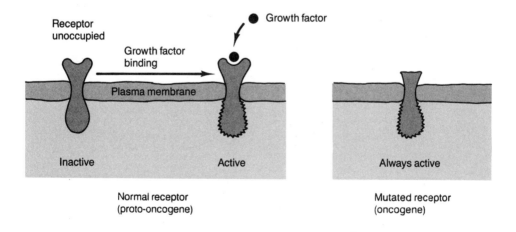

Figure 7.2

Conversion of a growth-factor receptor to an oncogene. The normal growth-factor receptor is activated by growth-factor binding. In contrast, the mutated receptor—an oncogene—is active even in the absence of growth-factor stimulation.

Table 7.1
ONCOGENES IN HUMAN TUMORS

Oncogene	Types of Cancer
abl	Chronic myelogenous leukemia, acute lymphocytic leukemia
bcl-2	Follicular B-cell lymphoma
bcl-3	Chronic B-cell leukemia
can	Acute nonlymphocytic leukemia
E2A	Acute lymphocytic leukemia
*erb*B-2	Breast and ovarian cancers
gip	Adrenal cortical and ovarian cancers
gli	Glioblastoma
gsp	Pituitary tumors
hox-11	Acute lymphocytic leukemia
lyl	Acute lymphocytic leukemia
c-*myc*	Burkitt's and other B-cell lymphomas, breast and lung cancers
L-*myc*	Lung cancer
N-*myc*	Neuroblastoma, lung cancer
RAR	Acute promyelocytic leukemia
*ras*H	Thyroid cancer
*ras*K	Colon, lung, pancreatic, and thyroid cancers
*ras*N	Acute myelocytic and lymphocytic leukemias, thyroid cancer
ret	Thyroid cancer
rhom	Acute lymphocytic leukemia
scl	Acute stem cell leukemia
tan	Acute lymphocytic leukemia
trk	Thyroid cancer

TUMOR SUPPRESSOR GENES

The other class of genes that are important in tumor development, the tumor suppressor genes, represent the opposite side of the coin of cell growth control. Whereas oncogenes stimulate cell division and tumor development, tumor suppressor genes normally act to inhibit these processes. If oncogenes are viewed as gas pedals, acting to accelerate the growth of cancer cells, tumor suppressor genes can be viewed as brakes, acting to slow down cell growth. In many tumors, mutations lead to the loss or inactivation of tumor suppressor genes, thereby eliminating the inhibitors of cell proliferation. The formation of oncogenes and the inactivation of tumor suppressor genes thus represent complementary events in the development of cancer, both contributing to increased cell division and loss of normal growth control.

Tumor suppressor genes were discovered more recently than oncogenes, so scientists currently know less about them. However, about a dozen tumor suppressor genes now appear to be involved in human cancers, and since this is a very active area of research, new tumor suppressor genes are rapidly being identified and analyzed. At least some of these genes, as might be expected, normally act in the regulatory pathways that inhibit cell proliferation. As discussed in chapter 3, normal cells are regulated by signals that inhibit as well as stimulate their growth, and it appears that tumor suppressor genes may be involved in such growth inhibitory signaling mechanisms. The inactivation of these genes therefore leads to the failure of a cell to respond to growth inhibitory signals, resulting, like the action of oncogenes, in uncontrolled cell division (Fig. 7.3).

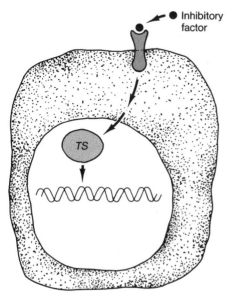

Inhibitory factor

TS

Cell division inhibited

Figure 7.3

Action of tumor suppressor genes. A growth inhibitory factor binds to a cell-surface receptor and stimulates the activity of a tumor suppressor (TS) gene product. The TS gene product then acts to block cell proliferation.

Oncogenes and tumor suppressor genes have thus been called the yin and yang of cell-growth control, the former acting to stimulate and the latter acting to inhibit cell proliferation. Not only do these two sets of genes have opposing effects on the cell, but they also may interact directly with each other. For example, some tumor suppressor genes act to inhibit the expression or function of oncogenes. Consequently, inactivation of these tumor suppressor genes leads to excess activity of the corresponding oncogenes, which then act to stimulate cell division. Conversely, several viruses, including the human papillomaviruses discussed in chapter 5, act by inhibiting the function of tumor suppressor genes. The control of cell growth is thus carefully balanced between stimulatory and inhibitory elements; abnormalities to either can tip the scale between normal cell proliferation and the uncontrolled growth of tumor cells.

The mutations leading to inactivation of tumor suppressor genes, like those resulting in the formation of oncogenes, most frequently occur only in single cells of the body rather than being inherited. However, some mutations in tumor suppressor genes are directly transmitted from parent to child, and mutations in these genes are responsible for many of the rare, inherited cancers discussed in chapter 6. For example, retinoblastoma, the childhood eye tumor, results from inactivation of the tumor suppressor gene called *RB*. In inherited retinoblastoma, mutations in the *RB* gene are transmitted from parent to child. In contrast, in sporadic, noninherited retinoblastoma, the mutations in *RB* occur only in the retinal cells that give rise to the tumor. Mutations in different tumor suppressor genes are responsible for other inherited cancers discussed in chapter 6, including Wilms' tumor (childhood kidney cancer), familial adenomatous polyposis (inherited colon cancer), and the multiple types of tumors associated with Li-Fraumeni family cancer syndrome (including breast cancers, brain tumors, sarcomas, and leukemias).

Most frequently, however, mutations of tumor suppressor genes are not inherited, instead occurring only in the cells that eventually become cancerous. Like oncogenes, mutations of tumor suppressor genes are important in many different types of tumors (Table 7.2). For example, although inherited mutations in the *RB* tumor suppressor gene are associated with a childhood eye tumor that is rare, the same gene is also involved in some of the most common cancers of adults. In particular, mutations of the *RB* gene appear to play a role in cancers of the bladder, breast, lung, and prostate. But the tumor suppressor gene most frequently involved in human cancers is called *p53*. It is responsible not only for inheritance of the Li-Fraumeni cancer family syndrome, but is also involved in a wide spectrum of common adult cancers, including those of the lung, breast, colon, and liver, as well as leukemias and lym-

Table 7.2
TUMOR SUPPRESSOR GENES IN HUMAN TUMORS

Tumor Suppressor Gene	Types of Cancer
APC	Colon/rectum cancer
DCC	Colon/rectum cancer
MCC	Colon/rectum cancer
NF-1	Neurofibrosarcomas
p53	Brain tumors, breast, colon/rectum, esophageal, liver, and lung cancers, osteosarcomas, rhabdomyosarcomas, leukemias, and lymphomas
RB	Retinoblastoma, osteosarcoma, rhabdomyosarcoma, bladder, breast, lung, and prostate cancers
WT-1	Wilms' tumor

phomas. All told, mutations in the *p53* gene may be involved in up to 50 percent of all cancers in the United States, so it is clearly a tumor suppressor gene of critical importance.

MULTIPLE GENETIC CHANGES CONTRIBUTE TO CANCER DEVELOPMENT

As discussed in chapter 2, the development of cancer is a gradual process in which normal cells become malignant through a series of progressive alterations. Cancers arise from single cells that have begun to proliferate abnormally. Progression to malignancy then occurs as the tumor cells undergo a series of mutations, leading to the acquisition of increased cell proliferation, invasiveness, and metastatic potential. Both oncogenes and tumor suppressor genes play important roles in the development of malignancy, and multiple mutations, affecting both types of genes, are usually required to result in the loss of growth control characteristic of fully malignant cancer cells. Some oncogenes and tumor suppressor genes are involved in the initial conversion of a normal cell to abnormal growth, whereas others play a role in later stages of progression to malignancy.

The *ras* genes, for example, can be converted to oncogenes as a result of mutations caused by a number of carcinogens, including some of the chemicals in tobacco smoke and ultraviolet radiation from sunlight. Mutations in *ras* genes appear to be very early events in the development of several types of human cancer, including those of the colon, rectum, and thyroid, as well as some types of leukemia. In these tumors, *ras* oncogenes are active in lesions representing early, premalignant stages of disease, for example, benign colon adenomas. Thus, *ras* genes are frequently mutated early in the process of tumor development—in at least some cases, probably by direct action of the carcinogenic agent involved.

The *p53* tumor suppressor gene also appears to be a direct target for mutations induced by environmental carcinogens. In this case, the clearest example is from studies of mutations that occur to the *p53* gene in liver cancers. Aflatoxin, in addition to infection with hepatitis B virus, is a major risk factor for liver cancer in southern Africa and China. As discussed in chapter 4, aflatoxin is a highly potent and very mutagenic liver carcinogen that may be present in contaminated supplies of peanuts and grains. Studies of liver cancers in patients exposed to aflatoxin have shown that they frequently contain mutated *p53* genes. Importantly, detailed analysis of these genes further indicated that their mutations were specifically induced by aflatoxin. Thus, the *p53* tumor suppressor gene is a direct target for mutations induced by this dietary carcinogen.

In other cases, oncogenes are involved in late stages of tumor progression rather than the initial stages of tumor development. Neuroblastoma, a childhood tumor of embryonic nerve cells, has provided the prototypical example of such a relationship. Neuroblastomas are commonly divided into four clinical stages, based on tumor size and the extent to which the tumor has spread from its site of origin (Table 7.3). An oncogene called N-*myc* is frequently active in more advanced stage III and stage IV tumors, but only rarely in stage I and stage II tumors. In addition, the behavior of individual neuroblastomas is closely correlated with N-*myc* activity. For example, those stage II tumors with active N-*myc* oncogenes have a much greater likelihood of further progression and

Table 7.3
ACTIVATION OF N-*MYC* IN NEUROBLASTOMAS

Stage	Description	N-*myc* Activation (percent of tumors)
I	Tumor confined to organ of origin	<10
II	Tumor extending beyond organ of origin but not crossing the body midline	12
III	Tumor extending beyond midline	65
IV	Widespread disease	48

Data from R.C. Seeger et al., Association of multiple copies of the N-*myc* oncogene with rapid progression of neuroblastomas, *N. Engl. J. Med.* 313: 1111–1116, 1985.

metastasis than do stage II tumors lacking N-*myc* activity. Similarly, stage III and IV tumors containing active N-*myc* genes progress more rapidly than those that do not. The N-*myc* oncogene thus appears to play a critical role in the progression of neuroblastomas, closely correlating with the development of increasing malignancy. In fact, whether a neuroblastoma contains an active N-*myc* oncogene is now considered a significant piece of diagnostic information. If so, it indicates a more rapidly progressing tumor and suggests the use of more aggressive treatments.

Activity of another oncogene, called *erb*B-2, appears to be similarly correlated with the malignancy of breast and ovarian cancers. Active *erb*B-2 genes are found in 25 to 30 percent of tumors of both types. In both cases, those tumors with active *erb*B-2 genes are more aggressive than those without. For example, in one detailed study, the average survival time for patients with ovarian cancer was approximately five years if their tumors did not contain active *erb*B-2 genes, but less than one year in cases where *erb*B-2 oncogenes displayed high levels of activity. Similarly, in breast cancers, *erb*B-2 activity is more frequent in advanced-stage tumors, and correlates with reduced survival.

Not only do oncogenes and tumor suppressor genes contribute to different stages of tumor initiation and progression, but the development of many types of cancer involves an accumulation of mutations in more than one gene of both types. The development of Burkitt's lymphoma provides a good example of the sequential roles of oncogenes and tumor suppressor genes in tumor development (Fig. 7.4). As discussed in chapter 5, these lymphomas are common in Africa, where they are initially caused by infection with Epstein-Barr virus. This virus carries its own oncogene, which acts to induce abnormal growth of infected lymphocytes. However, infection with Epstein-Barr virus is not by itself sufficient to produce a malignancy. Indeed, infection with this virus usually either produces no disease at all or causes mononucleosis. It thus appears that additional events, beyond the action of the viral oncogene, are necessary to cause a lymphoma. One such event is the activation of a cellular oncogene called c-*myc*, which drives the virus-infected lymphocytes further along the pathway to a malignant lymphoma. The *p53* tumor suppressor gene is also frequently mutated in Burkitt's lymphomas, indicating that it, too, plays a role in tumor development. Thus, the action of the Epstein-Barr virus oncogene is only the first step in lymphoma progression, with later steps involving at least one additional oncogene and a tumor suppressor gene.

Colon and rectum cancers were discussed in chapter 2 to illustrate the multiple stages involved in the development of a common human malignancy. These tumors also serve as the best example of the roles played by multiple genetic alterations. Colon cancers frequently involve

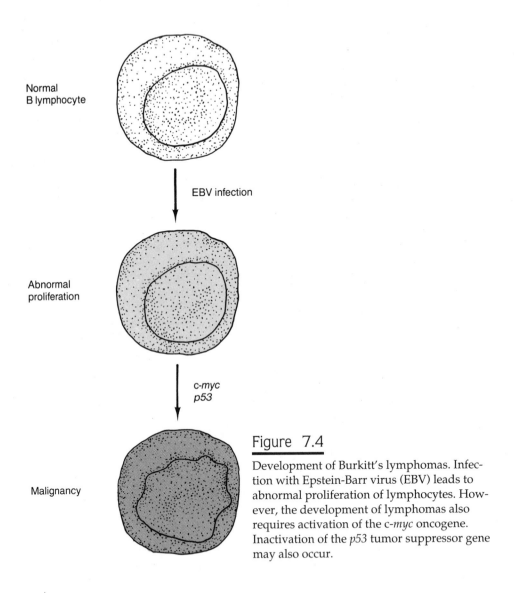

Normal
B lymphocyte

EBV infection

Abnormal
proliferation

c-*myc*
p53

Malignancy

Figure 7.4

Development of Burkitt's lymphomas. Infection with Epstein-Barr virus (EBV) leads to abnormal proliferation of lymphocytes. However, the development of lymphomas also requires activation of the c-*myc* oncogene. Inactivation of the *p53* tumor suppressor gene may also occur.

Figure 7.5 →

Oncogenes and tumor suppressor genes in the development of colon cancers. The *APC*, *DCC*, *MCC*, and *p53* tumor suppressor genes and the *ras*K oncogene appear to be involved most frequently in the indicated stages of colon cancer development.

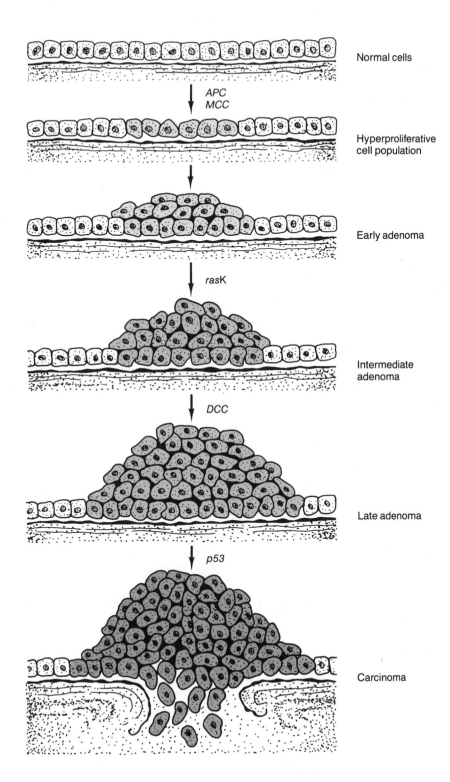

Normal cells

APC
MCC

Hyperproliferative
cell population

Early adenoma

rasK

Intermediate
adenoma

DCC

Late adenoma

p53

Carcinoma

mutations of *ras* genes as well as inactivation of four distinct tumor suppressor genes—*APC*, *DCC*, *MCC*, and *p53*. Lesions representing different stages of colon cancer development are regularly obtained as surgical specimens, so it has been possible to correlate these genetic alterations with discrete stages of tumor progression (Fig. 7.5). Such studies indicate that inactivation of the *APC* and *MCC* tumor suppressor genes are early events in tumor development. In addition, *ras* oncogenes are frequently found in premalignant adenomas, and thus appear to be involved in early stages of tumor formation. In contrast, inactivation of the *DCC* and *p53* tumor suppressor genes usually occurs at later stages of tumor progression. Mutations in these genes are only rarely found in early-stage adenomas but are frequently present in advanced adenomas and malignant carcinomas. In colon cancers, then, the *DCC* and *p53* tumor suppressor genes appear to be involved in later stages of progression to malignancy rather than in the initial stages of tumor formation.

Similar roles for multiple oncogenes and tumor suppressor genes very likely apply to the development of other human cancers, many of which have been found to involve defects in more than one gene. The development of human breast cancers, for example, may involve inactivation of two distinct tumor suppressor genes, as well as the action of two oncogenes, including the *erb*B-2 gene discussed above. Similarly, lung cancers may involve inactivation of three tumor suppressor genes as well as mutations of *ras* genes. The precise roles of these genes in tumor development are not yet understood, but the general correlation between tumor progression and accumulated mutations in both oncogenes and tumor suppressor genes appears to be applicable to a broad range of human malignancies.

SUMMARY

The uncontrolled growth of cancer cells is a result of mutations in genes that regulate normal cell proliferation. Two distinct classes of such genes have been identified: oncogenes and tumor suppressor genes. Oncogenes are mutated versions of genes that normally stimulate cell proliferation; their unregulated activity leads to abnormal cell growth and the development of cancer. Tumor suppressor genes, on the other hand, normally act to inhibit cell division, and their inactivation leads to a failure to respond to growth inhibitory signals. Oncogenes and tumor suppressor genes thus play complementary roles in control of cell growth, and mutations in both types of genes contribute to tumor development.

At least twenty different oncogenes and a dozen different tumor suppressor genes are involved in various types of human cancers. In rare, inherited cancers, mutations in tumor suppressor genes are genetically transmitted from parent to child. In the majority of cases, however, mutations in oncogenes and tumor suppressor genes are not inherited—rather, they occur only in the cells that eventually give rise to a tumor. Such mutations can result from errors that occassionally occur during normal cell division, or they can be induced by environmental carcinogens. In addition, cancer-causing viruses can introduce their own oncogenes into infected cells. Chemical, radiation, and viral carcinogens therefore share a common mode of action in their effects on the genes that control cell behavior. Multiple mutations, affecting both oncogenes and tumor suppressor genes, are required to result in the loss of growth control characteristic of cancer cells, and it is the accumulation of such mutations that is responsible for the progressive growth and spread of malignant tumors.

PART III

Cancer Prevention and Treatment

Chapter 8

Prospects for Cancer Prevention

As discussed in the preceding chapter, cancers develop as the result of accumulated damage to critical cell regulatory genes. Genetic damage occurs throughout life, and in some cases is unavoidable. For example, mutations sometimes arise as a consequence of errors made during the normal replication of DNA in dividing cells. In addition, some chemicals that react with DNA to induce mutations are formed as a result of normal cellular metabolism. There is, therefore, a "background level" of ongoing mutation that cannot be prevented and that, presumably, contributes to cancer development.

In addition, however, an individual's risk of developing cancer is affected by exposure to environmental agents. As discussed in chapter 4, it has been estimated that environmental carcinogens constitute risk factors for up to 80 percent of human cancers. In principle, then, much of the cancer problem could be eliminated by avoiding exposure to carcinogenic agents, which include chemicals, radiation, and viruses. This chapter will discuss the practical steps an individual can take, based on current knowledge, to lower his or her risk of developing cancer. Such steps include reducing or eliminating exposure to major known carcinogens and following good nutritional practices. The potentials and problems of additional means of cancer prevention will also be considered. These include the possibility of developing medications that prevent cancer, as well as continuing efforts to identify and eliminate synthetic chemical carcinogens from the environment.

SMOKING

The major identified cause of cancer, discussed in detail in chapter 4, is unquestionably cigarette smoking. Smoking is responsible for almost all lung cancer, and contributes as well to the development of several other types of malignancy. Tobacco smoke contains a number of carcinogens, which probably act both to induce mutations and to stimulate cell proliferation. Mutations in the *ras* oncogenes and in the *p53* tumor suppressor gene, which frequently contribute to the development of lung cancers (see chapter 7), may well result from the mutagenic activity of these carcinogens. In total, nearly one-third of all cancer deaths in the United States can be attributed to smoking.

Clearly, then, the single most effective action an individual can take to prevent cancer is not to smoke. Smoking pipes or cigars, or using smokeless tobacco (chewing tobacco or snuff), is less risky than smoking cigarettes. However, all of these forms of tobacco use are associated with substantially increased cancer risk, and, from the standpoint of cancer prevention, should be eliminated.

The risk associated with smoking was first widely publicized over twenty-five years ago, with the 1964 Report of the Surgeon General on Smoking and Health. It is now thoroughly established that smoking is not only a major cause of cancer, but also of heart disease, stroke, emphysema, and other respiratory diseases. The combined effect of all of these diseases is that 1 out of every 3 smokers will die from their habit. Such statistics make smoking the largest preventable cause of death in the United States. Nonetheless, over 50 million Americans, about one-third of the adult population, continue to smoke. Two to 3 million of these smokers are under the age of 18.

In the face of the striking risk associated with smoking, its continuing prevalence in our society seems surprising. Although individuals who have never smoked have the lowest risk of tobacco-related diseases, the risk of disease for smokers of all ages is substantially reduced by quitting. For example, as discussed in chapter 4, the risk of lung cancer steadily declines for exsmokers relative to those who continue smoking. Within about 20 years, the lung cancer risk for exsmokers becomes close to that of nonsmokers. In terms of overall life expectancy, it has been estimated that individuals who quit smoking before age 50 have one-half the risk of dying before age 65, compared to continuing smokers. Although quitting smoking is hard, it has major health benefits—both immediate and long term.

ALCOHOL

Excessive consumption of alcoholic beverages—more than four drinks a day—is associated with an increased risk of several cancers (see chapter 4). Cirrhosis, which can result from excess alcohol consumption, increases the risk of developing liver cancer, presumably as a result of chronic tissue damage leading to continuous cell proliferation. Alcohol is also a risk factor, particularly in combination with smoking, for cancers of the oral cavity, pharynx, larynx, and esophagus. In these cases, it is likely that the effect of alcohol is exerted primarily by potentiating the action of other carcinogens such as those present in tobacco. It is generally recommended that alcohol be used only in moderation—two or fewer drinks a day. Because of the combined effects of alcohol and smoking, minimizing alcohol consumption would appear to be especially important for smokers.

RADIATION

As also discussed in chapter 4, both ultraviolet and ionizing radiation, which act directly to cause mutations by damaging DNA, are risk factors for human cancer. Other kinds of radiation have also been discussed as potential carcinogens, including the electromagnetic fields generated by power lines and electrical equipment. Although the possibility of a relationship between electromagnetic fields and cancer incidence is still being investigated, the evidence supporting this association is generally not considered convincing. Likewise, radiation from appliances such as televisions, computers, and microwave ovens has not been associated with increased cancer risk. Most exposure to the forms of radiation that do cause cancer is from natural sources, some of which cannot be avoided. Exposure to some sources of potentially carcinogenic radiation can, however, be minimized as part of an individual's cancer prevention effort. These include sunlight, medical and dental x-rays, and radon gas in the home.

Solar ultraviolet radiation is a major cause of skin cancer, including melanoma. Mutations of both *ras* genes and the *p53* tumor suppressor gene (discussed in chapter 7) may be one mechanism by which ultraviolet radiation can lead to melanoma development. Fair-skinned individuals are the most sensitive. It is advisable to avoid excessive exposure to the sun, if necessary by wearing protective clothing and using a sunscreen.

As discussed in chapter 4, about 80 percent of ionizing radiation exposure is from natural sources, such as cosmic rays and radioactive substances in the earth's crust. Medical and dental x-rays constitute most of the remainder—nearly 20 percent—of an individual's total exposure to ionizing radiation in the United States. X-rays are now administered so as to minimize radiation exposure to both the patient and physician. The risk associated with these procedures is small, and is usually far outweighed by the resulting benefits. However, it is clearly advisable to avoid exposure to any x-rays that are not medically indicated.

Radon gas is a natural source of radiation (see chapter 4), which can be a significant source of exposure in the home. Levels of radon vary widely in homes throughout the United States, in some cases being high enough to impart an increased risk of lung cancer. The average level of radon in American homes is approximately 1.5 picocuries per liter of air, and the Environmental Protection Agency has recommended as safe a level of radon of no more than 4 picocuries per liter. About 7 percent of American homes (approximately 4 million), however, have radon levels in excess of this guideline. A small percentage of homes, but still numbering in the tens of thousands, have indoor radon levels in excess of 25 picocuries per liter, which corresponds to about a five-fold increase in lung cancer risk. As with other carcinogens that contribute to lung cancer, the risk of radon exposure combines with the risk of smoking. Thus, particularly for smokers, high levels of radon in the home can constitute a significant hazard. It is, therefore, advisable for people to monitor indoor radon levels in their homes and to take remedial action if indicated. Radon monitoring kits are obtainable in hardware stores, and the level of radon in a home can be reduced by sealing cracks in basement walls and floors or by increasing ventilation.

One area of public concern has been the potential increase in radiation exposure that might result from living in the vicinity of a nuclear power plant. Radiation pollution from these plants, however, appears to make an insignificant contribution to the natural level of radiation exposure, and several studies have shown that residents in the vicinity of nuclear installations do not suffer an increased cancer risk. This assessment, of course, refers to the radiation pollution that results from normal day-to-day operation of these plants. Concerns over nuclear safety with respect to the likelihood of accidents, such as those that occurred at the Three Mile Island (Pa.) Power Station in 1979 or, more disastrously, at the Chernobyl (USSR) Power Station in 1986, are obviously a different matter.

DIETARY FACTORS

The significance of diet to cancer risk was discussed in detail in chapter 4. Although it is commonly thought that dietary factors contribute to the development of a significant percentage of cancers, attempts to pinpoint the role of individual dietary components have been largely inconclusive. That is, the possible effects of specific dietary practices on cancer incidence are not firmly established. Nonetheless, general dietary recommendations to reduce cancer risk have been made by several organizations, including the National Academy of Sciences, the American Cancer Society, and the National Institutes of Health. These recommendations are in line with good overall nutritional practice, and may also help to reduce cancer risk. The basic dietary recommendations for cancer prevention are to (1) reduce consumption of high-fat and high-calorie foods, (2) increase consumption of fresh fruits, vegetables, and whole-grain breads and cereals, and (3) consume cured, pickled, and smoked foods only in moderation.

Obesity significantly increases the risk of cancer of the uterine endometrium, and to a lesser extent that of the breast. It is, therefore, advisable to maintain normal body weight, if necessary by restricting caloric intake. Recommended body weights for women are 100 pounds for 5 feet in height, with an additional 5 pounds per inch over that. Body weights 40 percent or more in excess of these recommended levels are clearly associated with increased risk of endometrial cancer, presumably resulting from excess stimulation of endometrial cell proliferation by the estrogen produced by fat cells.

High-fat diets have been linked to increased incidence of breast and, most convincingly, colon cancers. It is, therefore, advisable to reduce dietary fat intake. In the United States, fat constitutes approximately 37 percent of calories in the average diet, and may be greater than 45 percent for some individuals. Fat constitutes a much smaller proportion of dietary intake in countries with substantially lower rates of breast and colon cancers, in some cases corresponding to less than 20 percent of total calories. It has been recommended by a National Academy of Sciences committee that Americans reduce fat consumption to 30 percent of total calorie intake or less, which might be expected to reduce the incidence of colon cancer by as much as two-fold. The fat content of a variety of foods is summarized in Table 8.1. In general, a reduction in dietary fat can be achieved by eating more fruits and vegetables, utilizing lean meats, poultry, and fish, consuming low-fat dairy products, and eating fewer fried foods and bakery products.

Fruits and vegetables are not only low in dietary fat, but they also serve as rich sources, together with whole-grain breads and cereals, of several dietary components that appear to reduce cancer risk. These protective substances (discussed in chapter 4) include dietary fiber, β-carotene (a source of vitamin A), and vitamin C, as well as other compounds that appear to interfere with the action of some carcinogens. Some of the mechanisms by which these protective agents may act are discussed later in this chapter. It is important to note, however, that although diets rich in fruit and vegetables seem to be associated with decreased risk of some cancers, the importance (and perhaps the identity) of the individual cancer-protective agents in these foods is unknown. It is, therefore, recommended that individuals consume a *variety* of vitamin-rich vegetables and fruits, rather than relying on fiber,

Table 8.1
FAT CONTENT OF SELECTED FOODS

Food	Percent of Calories as Fat
Dairy products	
Whole milk	48
Low-fat milk (1%)	17
Butter	99
Cheddar cheese	70
Cottage cheese (low-fat)	18
Ice cream	47
Yogurt (low-fat)	8
Meats	
Ground beef (broiled)	64
Rib roast	53
Steak	56
Lamb (roasted)	39
Ham	61
Salami	68
Poultry	
Chicken (fried)	45
Chicken (roasted)	34
Turkey (roasted)	27
Seafood	
Flounder (baked, with butter)	45
Flounder (baked, without butter)	11
Shrimp (fried)	45
Shrimp (steamed)	9
Tuna (packed in oil)	38
Tuna (packed in water)	7
Baked Goods	
Cake	40
Cookies	54
Doughnuts	50
Fruits and Vegetables	nearly 0

vitamin, or mineral supplements. Moreover, some vitamins and minerals—including vitamin A and selenium—are toxic when taken in high amounts, so dietary supplementation with these agents can be dangerous. Whole-grain breads and cereals, as well as fruits and vegetables (especially beans and peas), are good sources of dietary fiber, which may serve to decrease the risk of colon cancer. Fruits and vegetables, especially citrus fruits and green and yellow vegetables, are also rich sources of vitamins A and C. Cruciferous vegetables (broccoli, Brussels sprouts, cabbage, cauliflower, collards, kale, mustard greens, rutabagas, turnips, and turnip greens) contain several additional compounds that may reduce cancer risk as well. Frequent consumption of a variety of these foods is generally recommended, from the standpoints of both cancer prevention and good general nutrition.

Finally, excessive consumption of smoked, cured, and pickled foods has been linked to increased risk of stomach and esophageal cancers. These foods contain nitrites, which can be converted to highly carcinogenic chemicals (*N*-nitrosamines) in the body. It is, therefore, generally recommended that these foods be consumed only in moderation.

OCCUPATIONAL AND MEDICINAL CARCINOGENS

Several occupations involve exposure to carcinogens in the workplace (Table 8.2). As industrial carcinogens have been identified, appropriate

Table 8.2
OCCUPATIONS ASSOCIATED WITH INCREASED CANCER RISK

Representative Occupations	Associated Cancer Risk
Chemical, dye, and rubber workers	Leukemia, bladder, lung, and liver cancer
Coal, gas, and petroleum workers	Bladder, lung, and skin cancer
Construction workers	Lung cancer
Furniture manufacturing	Nasal cancer
Leather workers	Nasal and bladder cancer
Metal workers	Lung cancer
Mustard gas workers	Lung, larynx, and nasal cancer
Nickel refining	Lung and nasal cancer
Underground miners	Lung cancer

Note: See Table 4.2 for identification of the carcinogens responsible for these occupational cancer risks.

regulatory actions have been taken to limit the exposure of workers to these agents. However, it is prudent for an individual to be aware of the potential carcinogenic hazards of his or her occupation, and to be sure to follow recommended safety practices such as wearing protective clothing or masks. Many industrial carcinogens, such as asbestos (see chapter 4), act in combination with smoking to impart a strikingly high risk of lung cancer. In many cases, therefore, simply not smoking substantially reduces the effects of industrial carcinogen exposure.

As discussed in chapter 4, many medicines are carcinogenic, but in most cases the benefit from treatment far outweighs the risk of cancer. For example, drugs used in organ transplant procedures are known to increase cancer incidence, presumably by suppressing the immune system, but the immediate need for treatment far outweighs the risk that these medications will act as carcinogens. From the standpoint of cancer prevention, the major medical treatment currently associated with increased cancer risk is postmenopausal estrogen therapy. Long-term administration of estrogen alone clearly increases the risk of cancer of the uterine endometrium. Thus, although postmenopausal estrogen therapy is beneficial to many women, the associated risk of cancer needs to be considered and discussed with a physician. Fortunately, it appears that this risk is minimized by treatment with low doses of estrogen in combination with progesterone, which counteracts the effect of estrogen on endometrial cell proliferation.

CANCER-CAUSING VIRUSES

As discussed in chapter 5, viruses are important risk factors for some human cancers. The viruses implicated to date as direct-acting human carcinogens are hepatitis B virus (liver cancer), papillomaviruses (cervical and other anogenital cancers), Epstein-Barr virus (Burkitt's and other lymphomas), and human T-cell leukemia virus (adult T-cell leukemia). As noted in chapter 7, these viruses act both by introducing their own oncogenes into infected cells and by interfering with the action of cellular tumor suppressor genes. Hepatitis B virus also causes chronic tissue damage, which may contribute to the development of liver cancer by stimulating excess cell proliferation. In addition, patients with AIDS have a high frequency of developing certain cancers, particularly lymphomas and Kaposi's sarcoma, as a secondary consequence of immunodeficiency. The causative agent of AIDS, HIV, is thus an indirect cause of an increasing number of cancers throughout the world.

The identification of a virus as a cause of cancer presents the possibility of developing a vaccine to prevent virus infection. Vaccines have been very successful in combating many viruses that cause serious human diseases, such as polio and smallpox, and may ultimately prove effective in preventing virus-induced cancers. The greatest progress in this area so far has been the development of a safe and effective vaccine against hepatitis B virus. The efficacy of this vaccine in cancer prevention is currently being tested in the Gambia, a small African country with a high incidence of hepatitis B virus infection and resulting liver cancer. Vaccination of children in the Gambia was initiated in 1986, and it appears that the program has been effective in reducing the incidence of virus infection. However, the effect of vaccination on cancer incidence will require long-term study. Since the lag time between virus infection and development of liver cancer is at least twenty to thirty years, the data needed to assess the effect of this vaccination program on cancer incidence will not be available until around 2010. Nonetheless, the use of vaccination to prevent infection with hepatitis B virus is very likely to have significant beneficial effects in reducing liver cancer incidence.

Although vaccination against other cancer-causing viruses is not yet available, steps can be taken to minimize the likelihood of virus infection. In the United States, the viruses of major concern are the papillomaviruses, hepatitis B virus, and HIV (cancers induced by either Epstein-Barr virus or human T-cell leukemia virus are rare in this country). Fortunately, none of these viruses is transmitted by casual contact, and there is no risk of acquiring cancer simply by exposure to an infected individual. The papillomaviruses, hepatitis B virus, and HIV are all sexually transmitted, so adherence to safe sexual practices is an important protective measure. Hepatitis B virus, as well as HIV, can be transmitted by contaminated blood products. Blood supplies used for transfusions are routinely screened to eliminate such viral contamination. However, it is critical for individuals to avoid other sources of contaminated blood, such as sharing needles used for intravenous drug injection.

THE POSSIBILITY OF CHEMOPREVENTION

As discussed above, several dietary constituents, such as fiber and certain vitamins, are thought to lower cancer risk. Evidence for the efficacy of any of these factors is not definitive, so it is currently recommended that individuals eat a balanced diet rather than relying on specific dietary supplements. However, the possibility of identifying or developing specific medications that would serve to reduce cancer risk, called chemoprevention, is an active area of cancer research.

Laboratory studies have identified hundreds of chemicals that appear to have some influence on reducing cancer risk in experimental animals.

These include the dietary agents suspected of lowering human cancer incidence (e.g., vitamins A and C), as well as many other compounds. Such chemopreventive agents seem to act by interfering either with the action of carcinogens—these are called blocking agents—or with the outgrowth of mutated cells—suppressing agents (Fig. 8.1).

Many blocking agents affect the metabolism of potentially carcinogenic chemicals, either by inhibiting the conversion of potential carcinogens to their active forms, or by accelerating the elimination of potential carcinogens from the body. Vitamins C and E, for example, can protect against stomach cancer by blocking the conversion of nitrites to carcino-

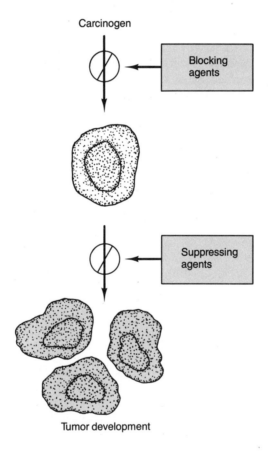

Figure 8.1

Actions of chemopreventive agents. Blocking agents interfere with the action of carcinogens, whereas suppressing agents inhibit the outgrowth of mutated cells.

genic *N*-nitrosamines in the digestive tract. Additional examples of blocking agents are the cancer-protective compounds present in cruciferous vegetables. These compounds stimulate the activity of enzymes in the liver and other tissues, which leads to the detoxification and elimination of a number of carcinogenic chemicals.

Other blocking agents may protect cells against the damage inflicted by carcinogens. Vitamin E and β-carotene, for example, protect cells against oxidative damage, which may contribute to carcinogenesis both by damaging DNA and by stimulating cell proliferation. More specifically, vitamin E and β-carotene are efficient scavengers of oxygen free radicals, which are highly reactive compounds inducing mutations in DNA and causing damage to several other cellular constituents. Oxygen free radicals are formed during normal cellular metabolism as well as generated within cells by chemical carcinogens and radiation. They may account for a substantial amount of natural and carcinogen-induced damage to DNA, so preventing this damage might significantly reduce rates of cancer development.

The other class of chemopreventive agents, suppressing agents, act to inhibit cell proliferation. The development of cancer requires proliferation of mutated cells. Agents that suppress cell proliferation might, therefore, interfere with early stages of the outgrowth of cells that have already sustained carcinogen-induced mutations. The chemopreventive agents that act in this way include vitamin A and related compounds (retinoids), tamoxifen (an estrogen antagonist), and calcium. Retinoids induce the differentiation of a variety of cells, concomitant with a decrease in their proliferation. Tamoxifen blocks the stimulation of breast and endometrial cell proliferation normally induced by estrogen, thereby inhibiting proliferation of these cell types. Calcium, likewise, acts to induce differentiation, and inhibit proliferation, of colon cells. In each of these cases, such suppression of cell proliferation apparently serves to prevent, or at least slow down, cancer development.

To date, the activities of these chemopreventive agents have primarily been demonstrated in experimental animals. However, studies are currently underway to determine the possible efficacy of several promising chemopreventive agents, including β-carotene, vitamin A, vitamin C, vitamin E, tamoxifen, and calcium, in humans. Moreover, encouraging results supporting the activity of retinoids in the prevention of cancers of the oral cavity, pharynx, and larynx have already been obtained. The primary risk factor for these cancers, like lung cancer, is the use of tobacco. Because of their usually heavy exposure to tobacco carcinogens, patients who have been successfully treated for one such cancer are at high risk of developing a second. But this risk was found to be substantially reduced (about five-fold) by administration of retinoids, although the high doses used in these studies also produced significant toxic side effects. A great deal of further work in this area is needed, but it is possible that, in the future, chemopreventive agents might be successfully employed to lower cancer risk.

THE QUESTIONABLE IMPORTANCE OF SYNTHETIC CHEMICALS IN THE ENVIRONMENT

Another strategy in cancer prevention has been the adoption of regulatory measures to eliminate carcinogens from the environment. The focus of this approach has been the identification, and subsequent elimination, of synthetic chemicals that cause cancer. At first sight, this makes good sense. An individual can do little to protect him- or herself against industrial pollution, so the possibility that carcinogens are being released into the environment clearly seems an appropriate area for government investigation and regulation. Indeed, such intervention has been of major importance in controlling the exposure of many workers to dangerous levels of occupational carcinogens. Environmental pollutants, however, are present in minute quantities compared to occupational carcinogens in the workplace, so hazards resulting from environmental pollution are less clear. The question of whether pollution with synthetic chemicals contributes significantly to cancer incidence is, in fact, highly controversial, as is the efficacy of attempting to identify and eliminate such low-level environmental carcinogens.

As discussed in chapter 4, many known occupational carcinogens are also present as pollutants in the environment at large. However, the levels of carcinogens in the environment are extremely low, so it is unlikely that these pollutants make any significant contribution to overall cancer incidence. The level of asbestos generally present in city air, for example, is more than 1000-fold less than that currently considered safe for occupational exposure. Even cases of chemical contamination from toxic waste sites, such as in the Love Canal (N.Y.) area, have not been associated with any apparent increase in cancer incidence.

Nonetheless, it can be argued that any exposure to a carcinogen might cause cancer and, therefore, should be prevented. The problem thus becomes one of risk assessment. How can carcinogenic pollutants be identified, and how can one determine the degree of hazard associated with such potential carcinogens?

The potential carcinogenicity of suspected chemicals is generally tested in mice or rats. In order to minimize the cost and the number of animals required for such tests, common practice is to administer a large amount of the suspected carcinogen. In fact, carcinogens are usually tested near the highest doses that are tolerated without severe toxicity, or the maximum tolerated dose. The significance of identifying carcinogens by this procedure has been seriously challenged by some scientists. First, these doses are sometimes hundreds of thousands of times higher than those to which humans are exposed. Second, more than half of both the synthetic and natural chemicals investigated have been found to cause cancer in animals when administered at the maximum tolerated dose. This is a surprisingly high fraction of chemicals to be carcinogens, and critics of the tests consider this to be a misleading result of the test procedure. The concern is that, since tested agents are administered at very high, near-toxic doses, cancers may result from the increased cell proliferation required to repair the chronic tissue damage caused by the test substance. Since such excess cell proliferation can clearly contribute, by itself, to tumor development (e.g., in liver cancer associated with cirrhosis), it is possible that this accounts for much of the carcinogenicity observed in these assays. If so, the induction of cancer by many of the suspected chemicals may be an artifact of high dose toxicity, which would be meaningless in terms of the lower doses to which humans are exposed. On the other hand, supporters of these assays argue that the mechanism of carcinogenicity of the tested agents is not known. Therefore, it is unwarranted to assume that positive results are misleading.

Even if one grants that high-dose carcinogenicity in mice and rats can be extrapolated to humans, is it likely that much lower doses can contribute significantly to cancer? And, does it make sense to eliminate chemicals from the environment on the basis of high-dose carcinogenicity in animal tests? One way to address these questions is to estimate what fraction of carcinogen exposure comes from the synthetic chemicals that are the targets of screening and elimination programs. An illustrative example is concern over contamination of vegetables with synthetic pesticides, including DDT, and other industrial pollutants, such as polychlorinated biphenyls (PCBs). A basis for comparison is the fact that all plants contain a number of natural pesticides to protect themselves from insects. High doses of about half of these natural pesticides, like the synthetic ones, are carcinogenic in mice and rats. In addition, the amount of natural plant pesticides consumed by Americans has been estimated to be more than 1000 times higher than the amount of synthetic pesticides consumed as a result of residual contamination. Thus, synthetic pesticides appear to make an insignificant contribution to overall carcinogen intake. Moreover, in spite of their relatively high content of natural pesticides, consumption of vegetables has been clearly shown in dietary studies to lower, rather than raise, cancer incidence. In fact, some of the natural pesticides actually serve as chemopreventive agents, by blocking the activity of other, more potent, carcinogens. Thus, neither the relatively high levels of natural carcinogens in vegetables, nor the much lower levels of contaminating synthetic carcinogens, pose a risk from the standpoint of human cancer.

Finally, one must consider the relative risks and benefits associated with a suspected synthetic carcinogen. In many cases, the minimal risk associated with synthetic chemicals is dwarfed by the benefits they provide. This consideration applies to all the ways in which our society benefits from synthetic chemicals, but the point can be made by just focusing on risk/benefit in terms of cancer. As discussed above, the cancer risk associated with the contamination of fruits and vegetables by synthetic pesticides is very small. However, if pesticides were not used, fruits and vegetables would be more difficult to produce and, consequently, less widely available. Since consumption of fresh fruits and vegetables clearly lowers cancer risk, it seems likely that a ban on pesticides would be highly counterproductive to the prevention of cancer.

Another example is provided by the artificial sweetener saccharin. As discussed in chapter 4, high doses of saccharin—100 to 1000 times higher than the amounts consumed by humans—cause bladder cancer in rats. However, epidemiological studies have found no evidence that human consumption of saccharin is linked to increased bladder cancer risk. On the basis of the animal data, saccharin was temporarily banned, although this ban has since been lifted. One presumed consequence of banning saccharin would be the use of sugar in its place, which in some cases would be expected to contribute to obesity, an established risk factor for cancer of the uterine endometrium.

The identification and elimination of carcinogens from the environment are clearly potentially important undertakings. Caution must be exercised, however, in order to focus efforts on those agents that make a significant contribution to human cancer incidence. Attempts to eliminate potential carcinogens which are present at only minute levels in the environment are not likely to substantially reduce cancer risk. Moreover, the cost of such efforts may divert resources from more profitable avenues of cancer prevention, such as the elimination of smoking. In addition, as discussed above, attempts to remove all synthetic chemicals which are potential carcinogens may ultimately prove harmful, rather than beneficial, to public health. A balanced risk-assessment policy which considers the extent of human hazard associated with low level exposure to potential carcinogens is clearly needed. But how to arrive at such a policy remains a subject of disagreement among experts.

SUMMARY

Individuals can take several different steps to reduce cancer risk. Foremost among these is avoiding the use of tobacco, which would eliminate about 30 percent of all cancer deaths in the United States. In addition, it is possible to minimize exposure to other known carcinogens, such as alcoholic beverages, some sources of radiation, occupational and medicinal carcinogens, and cancer-causing viruses. A number of dietary factors may also influence cancer risk and, although the specific effect of these factors is not known, it is prudent to follow generally recommended dietary practices. In total, it is estimated that these steps might prevent up to 40 to 50 percent of cancers in this country. However, risk factors, and therefore preventive measures, for many cancers remain unknown. The possibility of chemoprevention holds promise for the future, and is currently being investigated. On the other hand, the identification and elimination of potential carcinogens present at low levels in the environment does not seem likely to significantly reduce cancer incidence.

Chapter 9

Early Detection and Diagnosis

The next best thing to the prevention of cancer is early detection. As discussed in chapters 2 and 7, cancers do not arise as fully developed malignancies. Instead, they develop gradually as the result of mutations in multiple genes. As these mutations accumulate, tumor cells progressively acquire the characteristics of malignancy: increased proliferative capacity, invasiveness, and metastatic potential.

The importance of early detection is due to this progressive nature of tumor development. Prior to metastasis, most cancers can be cured by localized treatments, such as surgery or radiotherapy. Premalignant tumors (e.g., colon adenomas) and cancers that have not yet invaded surrounding normal tissue (carcinomas *in situ*) are usually completely curable, frequently by relatively minor procedures. More extensive surgery, perhaps in combination with other therapeutic modalities such as radiation, is required for invasive cancers, but such relatively localized treatments are still effective as long as extensive spread of the cancer has not occurred. Once a cancer has metastasized to distant body sites, however, localized treatments are no longer sufficient and a cure becomes much less likely.

The early detection of cancer is thus critical to the outcome of the disease. If the earliest stages of cancer (e.g., carcinoma *in situ*) could be reliably detected, lethality would be prevented, often by comparatively minor treatment. Indeed, steps taken to detect such early stages of tumor development are referred to as secondary prevention. For some kinds of cancer, routine screening of healthy individuals, before any symptoms are evident, is an effective way to detect the earliest stages of tumor development and reduce mortality from the disease. Other kinds of cancer, however, cannot usually be diagnosed until later stages, when symptoms of the disease have begun to appear.

THE PAP SMEAR AND CERVICAL CANCER

The Pap smear, developed in the 1930s, is the most outstanding illustration of an effective screening program. It is estimated that regular screening by Pap smear would prevent over 90 percent of deaths from cervical cancer, and such screening is responsible for the fact that mortality from this disease has decreased 75 percent since 1940 (see chapter 1). As an early screening test, the Pap smear possesses several desirable features that account for its effectiveness.

First, the Pap smear is a safe, reliable, and inexpensive procedure that involves minimal discomfort. A physician simply scrapes a sample of cells from the cervix with a cotton swab or wooden spatula as part of a routine pelvic examination. The procedure is painless and free of risk. The sample is then smeared onto a microscope slide, fixed, stained, and examined for the presence of abnormal cells. Carcinoma *in situ*, as well as even earlier stages of tumor development (dysplasias), can reliably be detected by this analysis, and it costs less than $20.

Not only can early stages of cervical cancer be detected by the Pap smear, but the course of the disease makes such early detection highly beneficial to the patient. Cervical dysplasia and carcinoma *in situ* usually persist for several years before progressing to invasive cancer. Thus, regular screening by the Pap smear is quite likely to detect the disease before it becomes life-threatening. Moreover, dysplasias and carcinoma *in situ* can be easily treated by several methods, including minor local surgery, which are virtually 100 percent effective.

There is little question that the Pap smear provides highly effective protection against cervical cancer. In the United States in 1990, about 50,000 cases of cervical cancer were detected as *in situ* tumors, compared to 13,500 cases that were not detected until they had reached the invasive stage. Moreover, it is thought that regular Pap smears could have prevented the vast majority of the remaining invasive cancer cases, which still account for about 6,000 American deaths annually (approximately 2.5% of cancer deaths in women). The American Cancer Society recommends annual Pap smears starting at 18 years of age.

EARLY DETECTION OF BREAST CANCER

Breast cancer is the most frequent cancer in women, occurring with an incidence of 150,000 cases a year in the United States. It accounts for about 30 percent of all female cancers, striking about one in every ten women. The mortality from breast cancer is about 44,000 deaths annually, making it second only to lung cancer, with 50,000 deaths annually, as a leading cause of cancer death in American women.

The prognosis for breast cancer strongly depends on early detection of the disease (Fig. 9.1). Five-year survival rates are nearly 100 percent for carcinoma *in situ*, 90 percent for locally invasive cancer, 68 percent for cancer that has spread regionally, and only 18 percent for those cancers that have metastasized to distant body sites. Thus, it is apparent that

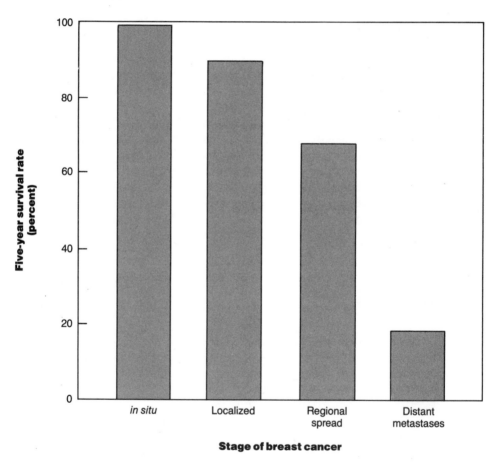

Figure 9.1

Survival rates following detection of different stages of breast cancer. Shown are five-year survival rates for patients diagnosed with carcinoma *in situ*; invasive cancer that is still localized to its site of origin; cancer that has spread to regional lymph nodes; and cancer that has already metastasized to distant body sites. (From American Cancer Society, *Cancer Facts and Figures*, 1990.)

screening procedures to detect early stages of breast cancer could have major public health benefits.

Three approaches to early detection of breast cancer are recommended by the American Cancer Society: (1) monthly breast self-examination, (2) an annual physical examination for women over age 40, and (3) mammography, as discussed below. Many abnormalities can be detected as changes or lumps in breast tissue, either during breast self-examination or by a physician. Any such abnormalities detected in self-examination should then be investigated by a physician to determine whether they represent development of a tumor. Even smaller breast lesions which cannot yet be felt can be detected by mammography, a low-dose x-ray of the breast. Thus, mammography has the potential of detecting breast cancer at the earliest stages of its development. As a cancer screening test, however, mammography has not achieved the wide success of the Pap smear, and in fact still remains a subject of some controversy.

Unfortunately, the clinical efficacy of mammography is not as great as that of the Pap smear, although there is convincing evidence that regular mammography can lower breast cancer mortality. Several studies have compared breast cancer mortality rates among women who receive regular mammography and those who do not. These studies all indicate that breast cancer death rates are reduced by about 25 to 30 percent as a result of screening with mammography and physical examination (Fig. 9.2). This is a significantly lower benefit than that derived from the Pap smear, which is thought to reduce cervical cancer death rates by over 90 percent. Nonetheless, given the high frequency of breast cancer, a 25 percent reduction in mortality would correspond to saving the lives of over 10,000 American women each year. From the standpoint of an individual woman in the United States, the lifetime risk of dying from breast cancer is approximately 4 percent. Regular mammography might reduce this risk to 3 percent or less.

Thus, although mammography is not likely to abolish breast cancer mortality, it does appear to confer significant benefits. These benefits must be weighed against potential risk, expense, and discomfort, all of which appear to be more significant drawbacks to mammography than to the Pap smear.

One concern that has been raised about mammography is the potential carcinogenic effect of regular x-irradiation of breast tissue. However, the x-ray doses used for mammography are now quite low, and the risk of developing mammography-induced breast cancers is negligible. For example, it has been estimated that mammography might induce, at most, one to five breast cancers among a group of 10,000 women screened yearly starting at age 40. However, approximately 1,000 of these women would be expected to develop breast cancer in the natural course of

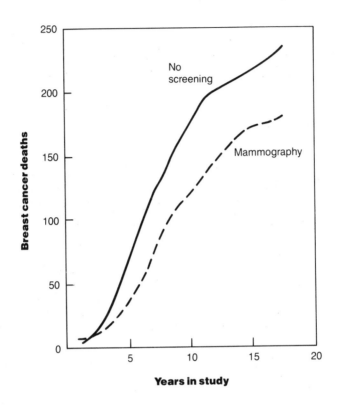

Figure 9.2

Effect of mammography on breast cancer mortality: the number of breast cancer deaths among women who participated in a study designed to evaluate the efficacy of screening by mammography. One group of women received regular mammography (designated *mammography*), while a comparable group of women had no regular screening tests (*no screening*). (From S. Shapiro, The status of breast cancer screening: A quarter century of research, *World J. Surg.* 13: 9–18, 1989.)

events. The increased risk of breast cancer resulting from mammography is less than 1 percent, which is clearly outweighed by the 25 to 30 percent reduction in breast cancer mortality as a result of early detection.

The other negative features of mammography are cost, discomfort, and the comparatively high frequency of false-positive test results. There is some discomfort from breast compression during mammography, but surveys indicate that most women find such discomfort only minor. The cost of mammography is relatively high, generally around $100 to $150. The frequency of false-positives, suspected lesions that are biopsied but ultimately do not turn out to be cancer, is about 80 percent. That is, only about 1 out of 5 biopsies performed following mammography reveals cancer. The problems arising from these false-positives, of course, are the performance of unnecessary biopsies, concommitant expense, and anxiety for the patients.

Nonetheless, it is generally felt that the demonstrated benefits of screening for breast cancer by mammography far outweigh its disadvantages. Consequently, the use of mammography as a regular program of breast cancer early detection, together with physical examination, is recommended by a number of organizations, including the American Cancer Society, the National Cancer Institute, and the American Medical Association. Their consensus guidelines for mammography screening are for women to have a baseline mammogram between ages 35 and 40, mammograms every one to two years from ages 40 to 50, and yearly mammograms at age 50 and over. Unfortunately, many physicians fail to recommend mammograms, which appears to significantly contribute to their underutilization.

SCREENING FOR COLORECTAL CANCER

Colorectal cancer is the third type of cancer for which early detection by screening is commonly recommended. Like breast cancer, colorectal cancer is extremely common, accounting for 155,000 cases and 61,000 deaths in the United States in 1990. In addition, as discussed extensively in chapters 2 and 7, colorectal cancers clearly develop in a gradual, progressive manner, and many of the steps in the development of these cancers have been identified. Furthermore, the benefits of treatment are much greater for patients with less advanced disease. For example, survival rates for patients with localized colon or rectum cancers are close to 90 and 80 percent, respectively. Survival rates drop to about 50 percent, however, for cancers that have spread to adjacent organs and lymph nodes, and survival rates for patients with distant metastases are only about 6 percent. Detection and treatment of precancerous lesions (adenomas) and early stage cancers could thus be expected to yield significant benefits.

Three approaches to the early detection of colorectal cancer are recommended by the American Cancer Society and other organizations: (1) digital rectal examination, (2) sigmoidoscopy, and (3) fecal occult blood testing. Each of these tests has different strengths and weaknesses. Their recommendation is further complicated by the fact that, in contrast to the situation with cervical and breast cancers, there are so far only limited studies demonstrating that screening for colorectal cancers actually reduces mortality from the disease. Existing studies do support the efficacy of screening, however, and further investigations are ongoing. Moreover, it is apparent that early detection can yield important benefits in the effectiveness of treatment. Screening for colorectal cancer is therefore currently recommended, even in the absence of final evidence conclusively establishing its effectiveness in reducing mortality.

Digital rectal examination is a simple test, which is easily performed as part of a routine physical exam. However, it is relatively insensitive as a screening test because only about 10 percent of colorectal tumors develop within the short portion of the rectum that can be reached by an examining finger. Therefore, although it should certainly be included in regular physical examinations, the effectiveness of the digital rectal exam for early detection of colorectal cancer is limited.

A significantly larger fraction of colorectal tumors can be detected by sigmoidoscopy, which is examination of the rectum and lower part of the colon with a thin, lighted tube. Using the most sensitive of these instruments, the flexible sigmoidoscope, it is possible to examine far enough up in the colon to detect about 50 percent of colorectal tumors. This is a significant improvement over the digital exam, but the drawback is a considerable degree of discomfort on the part of the patient. However, a recent study indicates that screening by flexible sigmoidoscopy could reduce mortality from colorectal cancer by at least 30 percent.

Screening for colorectal tumors by fecal occult blood testing has the potential advantage of detecting tumors in any part of the colon. The principle behind this test is that developing tumors cause minor bleeding, resulting in the presence of small amounts of blood, called occult blood, in the stool. To test for such small amounts of blood, a sample of stool is smeared on a slide impregnated with a chemical that changes color in the presence of hemoglobin. The stool sample can be obtained either at home or during a digital rectal exam, and the test is simple and easy to perform. Unfortunately, however, the occult blood test suffers from a high frequency of both false-negative and false-positive results. Many colorectal tumors do not release large enough amounts of blood to be detected. Rectal bleeding is often intermittent, so it is common practice to test multiple stool samples obtained over several days. Even when this is done, however, occult blood tests on 20 to 30 percent of patients with colon cancer are negative. The sensitivity of detection of premalignant adenomas and early cancers is still lower, probably about 50 percent. Thus, a high proportion of early colon cancers are not detected by this method. Conversely, occult blood tests are frequently positive in the absence of colon tumors. Such false-positives can be the result of bleeding from ulcers, fissures, or hemorrhoids. An additional source of false-positives is consumption of foods, such as red meat, that contain hemoglobin or other substances which react in the test. In any case, such incorrect results currently account for over 80 percent of positive occult blood tests. Nonetheless, any positive results must be followed up by further evaluations, which may include examination of the entire colon by colonoscopy or x-irradiation after a barium enema. Since these further tests entail a considerable degree of discomfort and expense, the high rate of false-positives is a significant problem in occult blood testing.

Despite these drawbacks, screening for colorectal cancer could have significant payoffs. As noted above, the actual reductions in mortality which result from current screening programs are not known, but such mortality reductions have been estimated to be about 30 percent. This would be similar to the effect of screening on breast cancer mortality. Since colorectal cancers are responsible for over 60,000 deaths per year in the United States, such a reduction in mortality from the disease would correspond to saving the lives of 20,000 Americans. In the absence of conclusive data, the American Cancer Society recommends (1) yearly digital rectal exams starting at age 40, (2) yearly fecal occult blood tests starting at age 50, and (3) sigmoidoscopy every three to five years starting at age 50.

EARLY DETECTION OF OTHER CANCERS

Several other cancers can be detected at early stages of disease during routine physical examinations. Consequently, an annual physical exam is recommended starting at age 40. Such annual physicals should include exams for cancer of the lymph nodes, oral cavity, skin, prostate, testes, ovaries, and thyroid, as well as tests for breast, cervical, and colorectal cancers discussed above. Prostate cancer can be detected by a digital rectal exam, a reason to recommend such an exam in addition to the possible detection of some rectal cancers. Additional procedures that are being evaluated for early detection of prostate cancer are ultrasound examination (described in a following section) and blood tests for prostate-specific antigen, a substance secreted into the blood by prostate cells. For women, pelvic exams are important for detection of uterine and ovarian cancers. Unfortunately, most ovarian cancers have already reached an advanced stage before they are detected in pelvic exams, so the possible use of more sensitive early-detection methods, such as ultrasound exams, are currently being explored. Early stages of oral cancers can frequently be detected visually during a medical or dental examination. Periodic self-examination is important for detection of skin cancers, including melanoma. Testicular cancers can also be detected by self-examination, as well as by a physician.

For many cancers, however, there are no available means to detect early stages of the disease before symptoms are evident. Unfortunately, this group includes lung cancer, for which there is no effective early-detection strategy. Periodic screening by chest x-ray is not recommended. Most lung cancers have already spread by the time they are large enough to be visualized in x-rays, so their detection by this method does not confer any significant advantage to the patient.

Early detection of cancer by screening, prior to the appearance of symptoms, is therefore an important—but not universally effective—step in reducing cancer mortality. In total, it is estimated that early detection could have prevented up to 50,000 American cancer deaths in 1990, approximately a 10 percent decrease in total cancer mortality.

SYMPTOMS OF CANCER

Those cancers that are not detected by screening prior to the development of symptoms still need to be diagnosed as early as possible to maximize the likelihood of a cure and the benefits of treatment. The American Cancer Society has called attention to seven early warning signals of cancer, which spell out the word *CAUTION*. Such symptoms do not necessarily indicate the presence of a cancer, but they should be investigated by a physician. Unfortunately, these symptoms are often not detected until the cancer has progressed to a relatively advanced stage. They are:

1. Change in bowel or bladder habits

2. A sore that does not heal

3. Unusual bleeding or discharge

4. Thickening or lump in a breast or elsewhere

5. Indigestion or difficulty in swallowing

6. Obvious change in a wart or mole

7. Nagging cough or hoarseness

DIAGNOSIS AND STAGING

When cancer is suspected, either because of positive results from a screening test or possible symptoms, further tests are undertaken to definitively diagnose the disease. The first step is a complete physical examination. In addition to palpation for abnormal tissue masses, the physical exam will include laboratory analysis of blood and urine. Microscopic examination of the cells present in blood can indicate the presence of leukemia, and other laboratory tests can provide clues to the presence of other cancers. For example, blood in the urine may be an indication of bladder cancer, just as blood in the stool may suggest colon cancer. Prostate cancers frequently produce substances—prostatic acid phosphatase and prostate-specific antigen—which can be detected in blood. The presence of abnormal immunoglobulins in blood or urine may signal multiple myeloma, a cancer of immunoglobulin-producing lymphocytes. High levels of certain hormones in blood may be indicative of cancers of hormone-producing cells, such as testicular cancers.

Other substances in blood may also serve as useful markers for some cancers, although they are not sufficiently specific or sensitive to form the basis of a definitive diagnosis. An example of such a tumor marker is carcinoembryonic antigen (CEA), which is a protein expressed on the surface of some cancer cells and some embryonic cell types. CEA is frequently secreted by colon and rectum carcinomas, but it is also produced by other cancers, including cancers of the breast, lung, and pancreas. Since CEA is usually only detectable in patients with advanced tumors, it is not a useful early diagnostic test. However, CEA is often used to follow the course of patients after treatment. For example, the detection of high levels of CEA following surgical removal of a colon cancer might indicate recurrence of the tumor or development of a metastastic lesion.

The next step in diagnosis, following a physical exam and blood tests, frequently involves visualization of any suspected tumor by x-rays or other imaging techniques. Imaging refers to a variety of noninvasive methods that can be used to view the inside of the body. In addition to conventional x-rays, a number of sophisticated imaging techniques are used for cancer diagnosis. Computed tomography—the CT or CAT scan—employs computer analysis of scanning x-ray images to generate cross-sectional pictures that portray a tumor's size and location much more accurately than conventional x-rays. This method is particularly useful for identifying and precisely locating abnormalities of internal organs, such as tumors within the abdomen. Nuclear magnetic resonance, or magnetic resonance imaging (MRI), is another technologically advanced imaging technique which, coupled with computer analysis, can provide extremely sensitive and precise information. It has the advantage of not using x-rays and, therefore, is not associated with exposure to carcinogenic radiation. MRI is particularly useful for analysis of tumors in tissues surrounded by bone, for example, tumors of the brain or spinal cord. Angiography is x-ray examination of the blood vessels, which may reveal distortions or the formation of new vessels indicative of the presence of a tumor. Radioisotope scanning methods permit detection of some lesions, including tumors in the liver, bone, brain, and thyroid gland, that cannot be visualized by x-rays. In this method, radioactive isotopes which concentrate in the target tissues are administered to the patient. Scanning for radioactivity can then detect abnormal patterns of isotope accumulation, allowing visualization of a tumor mass. Ultrasound is a technique in which high-frequency sound waves are directed at a part of the body. The "echoes" of these sound waves are then analysed, revealing the size, shape, and location of tissue masses. Ultrasound, like MRI, does not involve exposure to radiation. In addition, it has the advantage of being much less expensive than either a CT scan or MRI, both of which are costly procedures. Ultrasound can be used for visualization of tumors in a variety of sites, such as the stomach, pancreas, kidney, uterus, and ovary, although the image produced is not as clear as that obtained from a CT scan. Often, several different imaging methods will be used in combination to evaluate both a primary tumor and the possible extent of metastasis. These imaging methods are important not only in the detection of an abnormal tissue mass, but also in the precise location of a possibly malignant lesion for biopsy.

In addition to imaging, many tumors can be visualized directly by endoscopy, the use of a flexible, lighted tube to examine internal body cavities. Sigmoidoscopy, visualization of the lower part of the colon, was discussed above as a colon cancer screening procedure. Examination of the entire colon, colonoscopy, is not practical for screening asymptomatic individuals, but colonoscopy is performed diagnostically, for example, to determine the cause of positive results in a fecal occult blood test. Other internal organs which can be inspected directly by endoscopy include the esophagus, stomach, bladder, larynx, pharynx, bronchi, uterus, and ovaries. These procedures are of considerable value in the diagnosis of cancer, since they allow examination of internal organs without major surgery.

A definitive diagnosis of cancer ultimately requires a biopsy, so that cells in the suspected lesion can be examined directly by a pathologist. For leukemias, diagnosis involves examination of both blood samples and bone marrow biopsies. For solid tumors, a tissue sample is obtained by one of a number of techniques, depending on the type and location of the suspected lesion. Biopsy procedures range from removing a small sample of tissue with a needle, called aspiration and needle biopsies, to excising the entire abnormal tissue mass. Many potential tumors (e.g., breast tumors) can be biopsied externally, whereas biopsies of other tumors (e.g., colon tumors) can be obtained by endoscopy. Needle biopsies, coupled with sophisticated imaging techniques, are of considerable importance in cancer diagnosis, since these procedures allow tissue samples to be obtained from many suspected lesions without the need for major surgery. Tissue masses deep within the chest or abdomen, for example, can be successfully biopsied in this way.

Analysis of biopsy specimens will determine if a tumor is present, and, if so, whether it is benign or malignant. If a malignant tumor—cancer—is diagnosed, it is important to determine how far the malignancy has progressed. Particularly critical information in this regard is (1) the extent to which the tumor has invaded surrounding normal tissue, (2) whether the malignancy has spread to lymph nodes in the region of the tumor, and (3) whether the tumor has metastasized to distant body sites. As discussed in chapter 2, these factors determine the clinical stage of the tumor, which is of major importance in choosing an appropriate treatment strategy.

In additional to clinical staging, a number of other laboratory tests may provide information that is useful in predicting the course of disease and response to therapy. Tumor grading is based on the shape of the tumor cells and the fraction of tumor cells that are actively undergoing cell division. In general, more malignant cancers are characterized by abnormally shaped cells, large numbers of which are dividing.

It is also frequently useful to determine the DNA content and chromosomal composition of tumor cells. Abnormalities in amounts of cellular DNA and chromosome numbers usually indicate a less favorable prognosis, perhaps because they signal the accumulation of genetic abnormalities that occur during tumor progression (see chapter 7). In addition, specific chromosome abnormalities are diagnostic of some cancers. The prototype example is chronic myelogenous leukemia in which an oncogene (*abl*) is formed as a result of the transfer of DNA between two chromosomes (Fig. 9.3). The abnormal chromosome formed as a result of this

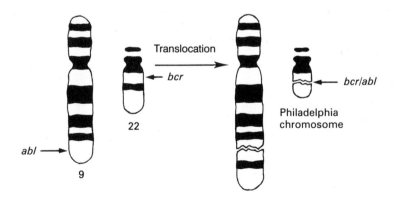

Figure 9.3

Chromosome rearrangement of the *abl* oncogene in chronic myelogenous leukemia. The *abl* oncogene is activated by a rearrangment that translocates it from its normal position on chromosome 9 into an abnormal locus (called *bcr*) on chromosome 22. The abnormal chromosome formed by this rearrangement is called the Philadelphia chromosome.

rearrangement is called the Philadelphia chromosome, after the city in which it was discovered. It is found in virtually all chronic myelogenous leukemias, and is therefore diagnostic of the disease. The expression of particular proteins may also provide a useful prognostic indicator for some types of cancer. In breast cancers, for example, expression of hormone receptors (i.e., estrogen and progesterone receptors) generally indicates a more favorable prognosis.

Direct analysis of abnormalities in oncogenes and tumor suppressor genes is also beginning to form part of the diagnostic picture for some cancers. For example, high levels of activity of the *erb*B-2 oncogene in breast cancers, or of the N-*myc* oncogene in neuroblastomas are indicative of more rapidly progressing tumors (see chapter 7) and may dictate more aggressive treatments. Detection of other oncogenes, such as the *abl* oncogene in chronic myelogenous leukemia, can also provide sensitive methods for monitoring the course of disease following treatment.

SUMMARY

Because of the progressive nature of the development of tumors, early detection and diagnosis are critical to the outcome of cancer. For some cancers, specific screening tests for healthy individuals are recommended, in order to detect the earliest possible stages of tumor development. The Pap smear, which is highly effective in detecting cervical cancer at a readily treatable stage, is an ideal example of such a screening method. Early screening tests are also recommended for detection of breast and colorectal cancers, although these screening tests (including mammography and fecal occult blood testing) are less effective than the Pap smear. Other cancers can be detected by self-examination, during routine physical exams, or by recognition of early disease symptoms. A number of further procedures are then used to investigate a suspected lesion, ultimately including a biopsy, to definitively determine whether cancer is present. If a diagnosis of cancer is made, clinical staging of the disease, together with other diagnostic assays, provide information essential to the choice of an appropriate treatment.

Chapter 10

Treatment of Cancer

Once cancer is diagnosed, a variety of possible treatment options are considered. The choice of treatment is determined by the type of cancer and the extent to which it has progressed. Substantial advances have been made in the treatment of some cancers, particularly childhood leukemias and lymphomas, which, in most cases, are now curable diseases. For most other types of cancer, however, the likelihood of a cure is highly dependent on detection of early stages of disease, before the cancer has spread from its site of origin. This chapter considers the current methods of cancer treatment, as well as some new—still experimental—treatment strategies.

SURGERY

Surgery is the first line of attack against most cancers. For benign tumors, surgical removal of the tumor mass results in a complete cure. The only benign tumors that are life-threatening are those that are inoperable because of their location, such as some brain tumors, or those that go untreated and become infected or compress vital structures as they increase in size.

For malignant tumors, however, the success of surgery depends on removing all of the cancer cells. If this is not accomplished, the remaining cells will continue to grow and metastasize even after removal of the bulk of the tumor. This is the reason early diagnosis is so important. Early-stage tumors (e.g., carcinomas *in situ*) that have not yet invaded surrounding normal tissue can be completely removed and are virtually 100 percent curable. Once invasion of adjacent normal tissues has begun, however, it becomes difficult to be sure that all of the cancer cells are eliminated by surgical removal of the tumor mass and immediately surrounding tissues. The extent of surgical removal of normal tissue around an invasive cancer is therefore highly dependent on the type of tumor and its extent of progression. In some cases, such as most skin cancers, it is sufficient to remove only the tumor and a small margin of surrounding normal tissue. In other cases, it is advisable to remove larger amounts of adjacent tissue, perhaps including regional lymph nodes to which the cancer may have spread, in order to eliminate all of the cancer cells.

Unfortunately, over 50 percent of cancers have already metastasized by the time of diagnosis and therefore cannot be cured by surgery alone. Nonetheless, surgical removal of the primary tumor plays an important role in treatment when done in combination with other therapeutic modalities discussed in subsequent sections of this chapter. First, the specimens of tumor and surrounding normal tissues, such as lymph nodes, obtained during surgery are of critical importance in determining the extent of tumor progression (clinical staging), and thereby designing an optimum strategy for further treatment. Even when a tumor has already metastasized, surgical removal of the primary tumor mass still, in some instances, forms an integral part of treatment, in combination with radiation and chemotherapy, for dealing with both local spread and distant metastasis. In addition to removal of a primary tumor mass, surgery can sometimes be used effectively to eliminate isolated metastatic tumors. And even in advanced cancer cases, appropriate surgical procedures, although not curative, may significantly reduce pain and other disease symptoms.

Thus, the role of surgery in cancer treatment is not confined to those cases in which the disease can be cured solely by removal of the primary tumor. However, surgery is ultimately a local treatment, the effectiveness of which is frequently defeated by the spread of tumors to regions that are too extensive for surgical removal (e.g., throughout entire organs), as well as by metastasis to distant body sites.

Even when successful, surgical removal of cancers can result in disfigurement or disablement. Such consequences often have profound emotional effects on both the patient and family members. Examples include radical head and neck surgery, loss of a breast from mastectomy, loss of bowel control from colostomy, amputation of a limb, loss of speech from laryngectomy, and impotence resulting from prostatectomy. Patients can often be assisted in dealing with these and other effects in a variety of ways, including breast prostheses, reconstructive surgery, artificial limbs, and use of mechanical or esophageal speech. A number of support groups, such as the Reach to Recovery, Laryngectomy Rehabilitation, and Ostomy Rehabilitation programs of the American Cancer Society, have been formed to help patients cope with these problems, which are discussed further in chapter 11.

RADIATION THERAPY

Radiation therapy, like surgery, is primarily a treatment for localized cancers. But it is an approach that can attack cancer cells that have spread through normal tissue beyond the scope of surgical removal. Thus, localized tumors are sometimes treated with radiation instead of surgery, and radiation is frequently used in combination with surgery to eliminate cancer cells that have invaded normal tissues surrounding the primary tumor site. In addition, some cancers are particularly sensitive to radiation, making it a preferential form of treatment for these diseases.

Previous chapters have discussed radiation as a cause of cancer, which induces mutations by damaging DNA. More extensive damage to DNA can kill cells altogether, which is the basis for the use of radiation in cancer therapy. Its effectiveness is limited, however, by the fact that radiation is not specific for cancer cells. It also kills normal cells and, consequently, can be highly toxic to the patient. (The problem of toxicity, resulting from an inability of a treatment to distinguish between cancer cells and normal cells, similarly limits the effectiveness of chemotherapy, as discussed in the next section of this chapter.)

A variety of types of radiation are used in cancer therapy, including x-rays, radiation produced by the decay of radioactive elements (e.g., cobalt), and beams of particles produced by linear accelerators (e.g., electrons). The radiation source is usually located outside the body, and a beam of radiation is directed at the tumor. In some cases, however, radiation is administered from an internal source; such as an implant of radioactive material placed directly in the vicinity of a tumor. Cervical cancers, for example, can be treated by implanting a capsule of radium within the cervix and upper vagina for a two- or three-day period.

As noted above, the primary action of radiation is to damage DNA. Such damage to genetic material is most lethal to cells that are rapidly dividing, so radiation selectively kills actively proliferating cells. Unfortunately, this includes normal cells as well as cancer cells. As discussed in previous chapters, several kinds of cells normally continue to divide throughout adult life. These include the blood-forming cells of the bone marrow, the cells that line the intestine, skin cells, the cells that form hair, and cells of the reproductive organs. The sensitivity of these normal cells is responsible for a number of side effects of radiation, which may include anemia, nausea, vomiting, diarrhea, skin damage, hair loss, and sterility. The extent of these side effects depends on the amount of radiation delivered and the area of the body that is irradiated. In some cases, radiation can be directed precisely at a tumor, with little damage to surrounding normal cells and minimal side effects. In other cases, sensitive normal tissues must be irradiated at the same time, limiting the amount of radiation an individual can receive during treatment.

Radiotherapy is sometimes a preferred alternative to surgery for curative treatment of localized tumors. An example is the use of radiotherapy for laryngeal cancer, where radiation provides effective treatment without the loss of speech that would result from surgical removal of the vocal cords. Similarly, radiation is used to treat some cancers in locations that are hard to treat by surgery. For example, skin cancers at sites like the eyelid or the tip of the nose may be treated by radiotherapy. Radiation may also be used instead of surgery for treatment of some cancers of the cervix, esophagus, and oral cavity. Hodgkin's disease, a form of lymphoma, is also effectively treated by radiation of the lymph nodes.

In addition to the use of radiotherapy as a primary mode of treatment, it is frequently used in combination with surgery to kill any tumor cells that remain after surgical removal of a primary tumor. In some cases, this is particularly useful in limiting the extent of surgery that needs to be performed. Early stages of breast cancer, for example, need no longer be treated by mastectomy. Instead, the generally recommended course of treatment is surgical removal of only the primary tumor and nearby lymph nodes, followed by radiation to kill remaining tumor cells. Some testicular cancers (seminomas) are also particularly sensitive to radiation, and are generally treated by limited surgery followed by radiotherapy of regional lymph nodes.

Radiation can thus be viewed as a localized cancer therapy that covers a broader area than surgery. In this context, radiation can extend the effective range of treatment of localized cancers by eliminating cancer cells that have spread from a primary tumor into surrounding normal tissues that cannot be completely removed by surgery. Tumors that have already metastasized to distant body sites, however, can no longer be treated by localized means, either surgery or radiotherapy, alone. Instead, treatment of these cancers requires the use of chemotherapy to reach cancer cells that have become disseminated throughout the body.

CHEMOTHERAPY

Although localized cancers can be effectively treated by surgery or radiotherapy, the success of these treatments is frequently limited by metastasis of cancer cells to distant body sites. Metastatic growths are often present by the time of diagnosis, although they may be too small to be detected. The existence of such metastases limits the success of localized treatment, necessitating the administration of chemotherapeutic drugs to attempt to kill tumor cells throughout the body.

Unfortunately, the drugs available for use in chemotherapy are not specific for cancer cells. Most chemotherapeutic agents act either by damaging DNA or by interfering with DNA synthesis. Thus, like radiation, they kill all rapidly dividing cells—not only cancer cells, but also the normal cells that are undergoing cell division, particularly those that line the intestine, blood-forming cells of the bone marrow, and cells that form hair. As is the case with radiation, the common side effects of chemotherapy result from the action of chemotherapeutic drugs on these normal cell populations. Damage to the lining of the intestine leads to nausea, vomiting, and diarrhea. The bone marrow is a site of major toxicity, since the loss of blood-forming cells causes anemia, ineffective blood clotting, and suppression of the immune system. Hair loss is also a common side effect of chemotherapy. Unlike radiation, chemotherapeutic drugs circulate throughout the body, so these toxic manifestations cannot be avoided. The effectiveness of chemotherapeutic drugs is thus limited by their toxicity, and the potential success of chemotherapy is determined by the relative sensitivities of cancer cells and normal cells to the drug being used. The goal is to kill all of the cancer cells while allowing sufficient numbers of normal cells to survive. The battle is fought by the administration of carefully regulated doses of the available drugs, and the physician attempts to walk a fine line between cancer cell death and normal cell survival.

A number of different drugs are used in cancer chemotherapy (Table 10.1), and these drugs act in several ways to inhibit cell division. One class of drugs, called antimetabolites, interferes with one or more steps in the synthesis of DNA. Since the genetic material must be duplicated each time a cell divides, these drugs block cell division, resulting in the death of actively proliferating cells. The antimetabolites used in cancer chemotherapy include compounds such as methotrexate, fluorouracil, cytosine arabinoside, mercaptopurine, thioguanine, and hydroxyurea. These agents act, either directly or indirectly, to inhibit the synthesis of DNA. Consequently, when DNA cannot be replicated, cell division is blocked and cells that are attempting to divide eventually die.

Other chemotherapeutic drugs act, like radiation, by damaging DNA directly. Also like radiation, the DNA damage induced by these drugs can sometimes contribute to the development of secondary cancers, particularly leukemias, in treated patients (see chapter 4). However, successful treatment of a patient's primary cancer is usually a much higher priority.

The largest group of DNA-damaging drugs are the alkylating agents, which react chemically with DNA molecules. Some of the alkylating agents used in cancer chemotherapy include mechlorethamine (nitrogen mustard), cyclophosphamide, melphalan, bischloroethylnitrosourea (BCNU), cyclohexylchloroethylnitrosourea (CCNU), thiotepa, chlorambucil, and procarbazine. These agents react directly with DNA to cause

Table 10.1
CHEMOTHERAPEUTIC DRUGS

Drug	Mechanism of Action
Actinomycin D	Inhibits RNA synthesis
Asparaginase	Degrades the amino acid asparagine in blood
Bischloroethylnitrosourea	Damages DNA
Bleomycin	Damages DNA
Chlorambucil	Damages DNA
Cisplatin	Damages DNA
Cyclohexylchloroethylnitrosourea	Damages DNA
Cyclophosphamide	Damages DNA
Cytosine arabinoside	Inhibits DNA synthesis
Daunomycin	Damages DNA
Doxorubicin	Damages DNA
Etoposide	Damages DNA
Fluorouracil	Inhibits DNA synthesis
Hydroxyurea	Inhibits DNA synthesis
Melphalan	Damages DNA
Mercaptopurine	Inhibits DNA synthesis
Methotrexate	Inhibits DNA synthesis
Mitomycin C	Damages DNA
Nitrogen mustard	Damages DNA
Procarbazine	Damages DNA
Taxol	Inhibits cell division
Teniposide	Damages DNA
Thioguanine	Inhibits DNA synthesis
Thiotepa	Damages DNA
Vinblastine	Inhibits cell division
Vincristine	Inhibits cell division

several types of damage, thereby blocking further DNA replication. Several other chemotherapeutic drugs, including bleomycin, cisplatin, mitomycin C, daunomycin, doxorubicin, etoposide (VP-16), and teniposide also act by damaging DNA molecules in different ways.

A few chemotherapeutic drugs interfere with cell division by inhibiting other cellular processes. Actinomycin D binds to DNA, but appears to act primarily by blocking gene expression rather than DNA replication. The agents vincristine and vinblastine block the process of cell division by inhibiting the movement of chromosomes. Taxol, a relatively new experimental drug isolated from the Pacific yew tree, acts in a similar manner. The enzyme asparaginase is used for therapy of acute leukemias. Asparaginase degrades the amino acid asparagine, which is essential for protein synthesis. Most cells synthesize their own asparagine, but many leukemic cells do not and, therefore, are dependent on obtaining asparagine as an essential nutrient from the blood supply. Asparaginase destroys asparagine in the blood and is, therefore, effective in blocking the growth of these leukemias.

The chemotherapeutic agents discussed above are only a representative list of those in use, and only a small fraction of the compounds that have been and are being tested for anticancer activity. Nonetheless, it is apparent that, in spite of the investigation of a large number of cancer chemotherapeutic agents, the cellular targets against which these drugs act are limited and not very specific for cancer cells. Most chemotherapeutic drugs either inhibit DNA synthesis, induce DNA damage, or otherwise block cell division. Therefore, the limiting factor in chemotherapy is the relative drug sensitivity of the cancer cells compared to the rapidly proliferating normal cells of the body. Some tumors are particularly drug sensitive and, therefore, can be successfully treated by chemotherapy. Often, these tumors are rapidly growing—and therefore most sensitive to DNA damage or inhibition of DNA synthesis—but the basis of selective toxicity to tumor cells versus normal cells is not well understood.

Notable examples of successes with chemotherapy include the treatment of Burkitt's lymphoma, Hodgkin's disease, acute lymphocytic leukemia, choriocarcinoma, and testicular cancer. Many other forms of cancer, however, including most common cancers of adults, are less responsive to chemotherapeutic drugs, which then become ineffective because the overwhelming toxic side effects prevent the administration of high enough doses to kill the cancer cells.

DRUG RESISTANCE AND COMBINATION CHEMOTHERAPY

As discussed above, the problem faced in chemotherapy is how to eradicate cancer cells while minimizing toxicity to normal cells. Since most chemotherapeutic agents have limited target specificity, the doses that can be employed must always represent a compromise between these two considerations, so complete elimination of tumor cells is a goal not easily attained. In addition, some cells in a cancer are frequently resistant to the action of any given drug and, therefore, survive treatment. Even if most of the cancer cells are killed, a small number of such drug-resistant survivors will grow back to form a tumor that no longer responds to the initial agent. The phenomenon of drug resistance thus poses a major problem to successful chemotherapy.

There are several ways in which cancer cells can become resistant to chemotherapeutic drugs, and the generation of drug-resistant cancer cells occurs frequently, in part as a result of the characteristic genetic instability of cancer cells (see chapter 3). Many different kinds of mutations can render cancer cells resistant to chemotherapeutic drugs. Tumor cells become resistant to methotrexate, for example, by making increased amounts of the target enzyme that methotrexate inhibits. Tolerable doses of methotrexate are then no longer effective, and DNA synthesis is able to proceed in the tumor cells. In other cases, cancer cells become drug-resistant as a result of mutations that make the tumor cells unable to take up the chemotherapeutic drugs, or convert them to their active forms inside the cells.

Not only do mutations render cancer cells resistant to single chemotherapeutic agents, but cancer cells sometimes become resistant to multiple different drugs at the same time. This phenomenon, known as multidrug resistance, is obviously particularly troublesome from the standpoint of chemotherapy. One form of multidrug resistance results from abnormally high expression of a cell surface protein that acts to "pump" a variety of chemotherapeutic drugs out of the cell before they can act. Normally, this protein serves to protect cells against potentially toxic foreign compounds. Its overexpression, however, renders cancer cells simultaneously resistant to several different chemotherapeutic drugs, including actinomycin D, daunomycin, doxorubicin, vinblastine, vincristine, mitomycin C, etoposide, and teniposide.

One approach to overcoming the problem posed by drug resistance is the administration of combinations of several different chemotherapeutic agents. The rationale is that, while many cancer cells may be resistant to one or even two drugs in combination, it is unlikely that any one cell will be resistant to all of the drugs being administered. Consequently, an appropriate combination of drugs has the theoretical potential of eradicating all cells in a tumor. Given the phenomenon of multidrug resistance, however, it is obviously important to choose a spectrum of drugs such that cancer cells do not become resistant to all drugs in a combination simultaneously.

Additional advantage is attained by using combinations of drugs with nonoverlapping patterns of toxicity to normal cells. An example is the use of doxorubicin, which is primarily toxic to the bone marrow, in combination with vincristine, which causes relatively little bone marrow toxicity. Such combinations allow the physician to maximize the antitumor effects of each drug, while remaining within the limits of toxicity tolerated by the patient.

The use of drug combinations is responsible for most of the progress that has been made in cancer chemotherapy over the last several decades. Single chemotherapeutic agents have only shown notable activity in the treatment of Burkitt's lymphoma (cyclophosphamide) and choriocarcinoma (methotrexate). Combinations of drugs, however, have resulted in successful treatment of several other kinds of cancer, including acute lymphocytic leukemia, Hodgkin's disease, non-Hodgkin's lymphoma, and testicular carcinoma. Testicular carcinoma, for example, is treated by combination chemotherapy with cisplatin, bleomycin, and etoposide. Unfortunately, however, curative chemotherapy for most common adult malignancies (e.g., breast, colon, and lung carcinomas) remains elusive.

BONE MARROW TRANSPLANTATION

As discussed above, the blood-forming cells of the bone marrow are one of the rapidly proliferating types of normal cells that, because of toxicity, limit the effectiveness of chemotherapy. Bone marrow transplantation is an attempt to bypass this toxicity, thereby allowing the use of much higher doses of drugs or radiation to eliminate tumor cells. In this procedure, the patient is treated with intensive, high doses of radiation or chemotherapy, which would normally be intolerable due to the destruction of blood-forming cells of the bone marrow. The patient is rescued following the conclusion of treatment, however, by receiving a transplant of new, healthy marrow. The cells within this donor marrow are able to repopulate and restore the blood-forming system of the patient, which ultimately regains normal function.

Bone marrow transplantation is most frequently used for treatment of leukemias and lymphomas, although it is also being evaluated as a possible therapy for some solid tumors. Usually, a normal tissue-matched donor provides the marrow that the patient receives after radiation or chemotherapy. In some cases, however, the patient's own bone marrow may be harvested before chemotherapy is initiated, stored, and then returned to the patient after chemotherapy has been completed. In these cases, the marrow must either be free of cancer cells at the time of harvest or treated to remove cancer cells before it is reintroduced into the patient.

Because of the high-dose chemotherapy used in this procedure, toxic effects, including nausea and vomiting, are severe. In addition, the patient's normal blood-cell and immune-system functions are suppressed until the donor bone marrow becomes fully active. Marrow function is usually restored in a period of two to four weeks, but it generally takes several months before the patient's immune system recovers full function. Because of the resulting high susceptibility to infection, patients are sometimes maintained in special rooms that are kept as free from infectious agents as possible. Other immunological complications, such as graft-versus-host disease, may also occur, so patients are intensively monitored both during hospitalization and for several months after being discharged.

HORMONE THERAPY

A hallmark of cancer cells is their failure to respond to the mechanisms that regulate normal cell proliferation. In many cancers, however, this lack of regulation is not complete, so proliferation of the cancer cells can still be modulated by some of the factors that control normal cell division. More specifically, some tumor cells are still responsive to the hormones that regulate proliferation of their normal counterparts. In these cases, manipulation of hormone levels can be an effective means of cancer treatment (Table 10.2).

As discussed in previous chapters, estrogen stimulates the proliferation of cells of both the breast and the uterine endometrium. Indeed, excess estrogen stimulation is associated with an increased risk of cancer at these sites. Conversely, interference with the hormonal pathways that drive normal cell proliferation can sometimes inhibit the proliferation of cancer cells. Breast cancers can be treated by interfering with estrogen-stimulated cell proliferation, for example, by administration of the anti-

Table 10.2
HORMONE THERAPIES

Type of Cancer	Hormone Treatment
Acute promyelocytic leukemia	Retinoic acid
Breast cancer	Tamoxifen
Endometrial cancer	Progesterone
Lymphocytic leukemia and lymphoma	Prednisone
Prostate cancer	Orchiectomy, estrogen, GnRH analogs, antiandrogens

estrogen tamoxifen. Tamoxifen is structurally similar to estrogen, but it acts to antagonize estrogen-induced processes, thereby inhibiting the growth of estrogen-dependent breast cancers. About 50 percent of patients with breast cancer, usually those whose tumors express detectable levels of estrogen receptor, respond to such treatment. Although tamoxifen produces some side effects, these are much less severe than those resulting from chemotherapeutic drugs that interfere with cell proliferation in a more general way.

The proliferation of uterine endometrial cells during the menstrual cycle is stimulated by estrogen and inhibited by progesterone. Thus, the most common hormone therapy for endometrial cancer is administration of synthetic progesterones to inhibit cell growth, a strategy that is successful in about one-third of patients. Antiestrogens, such as tamoxifen, may also be active against some endometrial cancers.

Prostate cancers are also hormone-responsive, in this case being stimulated by androgens such as testosterone. Hormone therapy is standard treatment to slow the growth of advanced prostate cancers that have spread through the body. Different strategies are employed, all with the goal of blocking androgen stimulation of the cancer cells (Fig. 10.1). First, since the testes are the primary source of androgens in the body, removal of the testicles (orchiectomy) may be recommended. Alternatively, the production of androgens can be inhibited by administration of other hormones. Androgen production in the testes is triggered by hormones, called gonadotropins, that are produced by the pituitary gland. Estrogens, for example diethylstilbestrol (DES), suppress the production of pituitary gonadotropins and, consequently, inhibit androgen synthesis in the testes. A similar effect is achieved by administration of analogs of gonadotropin-releasing hormone (GnRH). GnRH is a hormone produced by the hypothalamus that acts on the pituitary to signal gonadotropin release. Continuous administration of GnRH analogs, however, suppresses gonadotropin release, thereby inhibiting androgen synthesis. Finally, antiandrogens can act at the level of the prostate cancer cell itself, by blocking the binding of androgens to their receptor protein. Such hormone therapies are not curative, but they do significantly inhibit tumor progression, relieve pain, and prolong the lives of many patients.

Hormones produced by the adrenal gland, called adrenal glucocorticoids, inhibit the proliferation of lymphoid cells. Consequently, glucocorticoids (usually prednisone) are commonly employed in the treatment of leukemias and lymphomas, including acute lymphocytic leukemia, Hodgkin's disease, non-Hodgkin's lymphomas, and myeloma. A standard therapeutic regimen for Hodgkin's disease, for example, is the combination of two alkylating agents (mechlorethamine and procarbazine), vincristine, and prednisone.

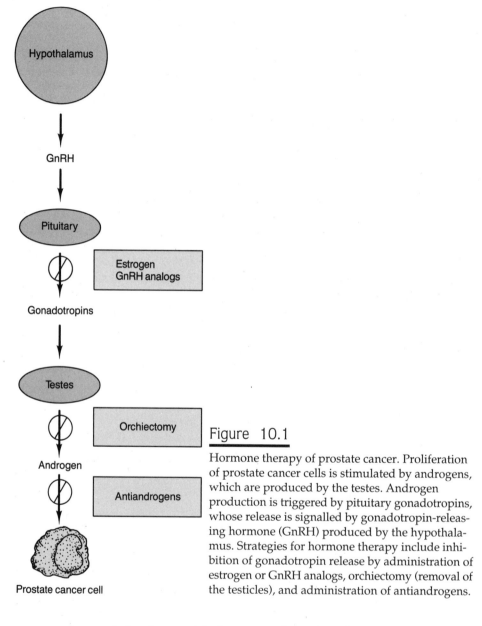

Figure 10.1

Hormone therapy of prostate cancer. Proliferation of prostate cancer cells is stimulated by androgens, which are produced by the testes. Androgen production is triggered by pituitary gonadotropins, whose release is signalled by gonadotropin-releasing hormone (GnRH) produced by the hypothalamus. Strategies for hormone therapy include inhibition of gonadotropin release by administration of estrogen or GnRH analogs, orchiectomy (removal of the testicles), and administration of antiandrogens.

A recent development in hormone therapy is the treatment of acute promyelocytic leukemia with retinoic acid (vitamin A). Retinoic acid induces these leukemic cells to differentiate, thus causing cessation of their proliferation. In view of the therapeutic activity of retinoic acid for acute promyelocytic leukemia, it is especially noteworthy that a mutated form of the retinoic acid receptor acts as an oncogene in this disease. In its mutated oncogene form, the receptor apparently acts to block normal differentiation, thereby contributing to the development of leukemia. However, further manipulation of its activity by administration of retinoic acid bypasses the block to differentiation and reverses the behavior of the leukemic cells. This is the first possible example of a direct relationship between an oncogene and a tumor treatment, although the possibility of directing therapies to specific oncogene targets is an area of active investigation in current cancer research (see chapter 15 for further discussion).

IMMUNOTHERAPY

Immunotherapy is the attempt to use the body's natural defense mechanism, the immune system, to fight cancer. The notion that the immune system does, in fact, provide a defense against cancer is supported by the fact that individuals with inherited or acquired immunodeficiencies suffer a high incidence of certain tumors (see chapters 4 to 6). It is noteworthy, however, that such immunodeficiencies particularly increase susceptibility to a few specific kinds of cancers, such as lymphomas, rather than to all cancers. Interestingly, too, the cancers that occur most frequently in immunodeficient individuals are those associated with tumor viruses (e.g., Epstein-Barr virus–induced lymphomas, discussed in chapter 5), suggesting that a normal immune response is particularly important as a defense against virus-induced tumors. However, immune reactions against a variety of other kinds of tumors also occur, so the immune system may provide a defense against tumor development in general.

The goal of immunotherapy, then, is to bolster the effectiveness of a patient's immune system in an attempt to eliminate cancer cells. Two general approaches are used: (1) nonspecific stimulation of the patient's own immune response, and (2) the administration of specific kinds of immune cells or secreted products that act against the patient's cancer cells.

Nonspecific stimulation of the immune system has usually been ineffective as a therapeutic strategy against most cancers in both humans and experimental animals. However, this approach has recently been found to yield significant benefits in the treatment of human colon cancer. The drug employed in this case is levamisole, which stimulates a variety of immune responses and inhibits the growth of some tumors in experimental animals. Based on these studies, treatment with levamisole and fluorouracil (an antimetabolite discussed above) in combination was tried as a postsurgical therapy for patients with colon cancers that had spread to regional lymph nodes. The five-year survival rate for these patients after surgery alone is less than 50 percent, due to metastases that are not eliminated by surgical removal of the primary tumor mass. Neither fluorouracil nor levamisole alone has a significant effect on this post-surgical prognosis. However, these two drugs in combination resulted in a reduction of about one-third in the rates of tumor recurrence and mortality following surgery. Although modest, this represents a clear benefit of postsurgical treatment with levamisole + fluorouracil over surgery alone. Consequently, this treatment modality has now been accepted as standard therapy for patients with lymph node–positive colon cancer.

In contrast to levamisole and other drugs that nonspecifically stimulate the patient's immune system, alternative modes of immunotherapy are specifically directed against the patient's tumor. An example of such a therapy, currently under clinical evaluation, is treatment with tumor-infiltrating lymphocytes. In this approach, large numbers of lymphocytes with antitumor reactivity are administered to the patient. These lymphocytes are obtained from surgically removed tumor specimens, grown to large cell numbers in the laboratory, and then transferred back to the patient, together with the growth factor interleukin-2, to further stimulate their proliferation and antitumor activity. The hope is that sufficiently large numbers of these antitumor lymphocytes will react effectively against the cancer. To date, such treatments have been most active in patients with advanced kidney cancers and melanoma, with positive responses being achieved in about 20 percent of such patients. Although far from a complete success, such a response rate is favorable compared to other treatments of these two tumor types. The results of these trials are, therefore, encouraging, and further studies are in progress.

Another variety of specific immunotherapy is the administration of monoclonal antibodies, which are antibodies produced by single clones of lymphocytes against a specific substance. Lymphocytes producing monoclonal antibodies can be generated and propagated in the laboratory, so that large quantities of these highly specific antibodies can be obtained. A number of monoclonal antibodies that react against proteins on the surface of cancer cells have been tried as therapeutic reagents, but this approach has not proven very successful. An alternative application, however, is the use of monoclonal antibodies to deliver drugs or sources of radiation specifically to tumor cells. For example, an antitumor antibody coupled to a radioactive isotope might serve to direct this source of radiation specifically to cancer cells, resulting in their selective eradication. Such applications of monoclonal antibodies in drug targeting are being actively studied.

Yet another variation in immunotherapy is the administration of factors secreted by lymphocytes, rather than administration of lymphocytes or antibodies per se. Such factors include interleukin-2, the interferons, and tumor necrosis factor. They may have both antiproliferative effects on tumor cells and immune stimulatory effects on the host. Interleukin-2 stimulates the activity of lymphocytes with antitumor activity. As noted above, it is utilized together with the transfer of tumor-infiltrating lymphocytes to maximize their antitumor effect. Interferon, the most thoroughly studied of the antitumor factors, appears to both stimulate the immune system of the host and to have direct effects on tumor cells. So far, interferon has shown activity against only a few human cancers, particularly certain leukemias, but further studies of the combined effects of interferon with other chemotherapeutic drugs are continuing. Tumor necrosis factor also has direct effects against tumor cells. Unfortunately, however, treatment with tumor necrosis factor also results in considerable toxic side effects, limiting its therapeutic effectiveness.

Thus, although immunotherapy offers the promise of a natural, and therefore potentially nontoxic, approach to cancer treatment, this promise has not yet been translated into widespread practice. Nonetheless, this is an active area of cancer research, and it is possible that further studies will provide more effective means of manipulating the immune system to target tumor cells for selective elimination.

CLINICAL TRIALS VERSUS UNPROVEN TREATMENTS

Several of the treatment modalities discussed in this chapter represent therapies that are still under investigation rather than having already been established as standard cancer treatments. Indeed, since cancer treatments are obviously less than entirely satisfactory today, new drugs and treatment protocols are continuously being developed.

The process of drug development is a painstaking one, which involves extensive laboratory and experimental animal studies of any new drug prior to its use in humans. On the average, it takes twelve years and $240 million for a pharmaceutical company to develop a successful new drug from conception to general use in medical practice. The process is closely regulated by the Food and Drug Administration (FDA), which must approve human use of any new drug based on its satisfactory performance in a series of required tests in animals. Only when a drug has shown significant antitumor activity with tolerable side effects in experimental animals is it finally ready to be tested in humans.

Once a new drug or treatment regimen is ready for human testing, known as clinical trial, it undergoes evaluation via a three stage process. At each stage, patients who volunteer to participate as subjects are informed of the possible risks and benefits. Phase I involves administration of the drug to a small number of advanced-cancer patients, usually about twenty, in order to determine how well the drug is tolerated by humans. If no prohibitive toxicity is encountered, the drug is tested in phase II trials on a larger group of advanced-cancer patients—perhaps up to a hundred—with an attempt to determine efficacy in different types of tumors. Patients asked to participate in either phase I or II trials are only advanced-cancer patients whose malignancies have failed to respond to standard treatments, so their participation in these tests does not interfere with conventional treatment, and has the possibility of beneficial effects. If a drug appears effective in phase II trials, it proceeds to phase III testing. These studies involve much larger numbers of patients (up to 1000 or more) who have earlier stages of a particular malignancy. In these trials, the test treatment is compared to the current standard treatment for the type of cancer being investigated, with subjects usually assigned randomly to receive either the standard or the experimental treatment. An example is the trial of levamisole + fluorouracil in colon cancer, which was discussed above. Approximately 1200 patients participated in this trial. They all received surgery, the standard treatment; and some then received follow-up treatment with levamisole + fluorouracil, the experimental treatment. Once the efficacy of this drug combination became apparent, postsurgical treatment with levamisole + fluorouracil was accepted as standard for future practice.

Many patients hesitate to participate in clinical trials for fear of being used as "guinea pigs." Clinical trials are indeed experimental, but without them no progress in the development of new drugs could be made. It is important to realize that a considerable amount of drug testing and review has already taken place by the clinical-trial stage, and that patients participating in such trials are not denied any treatment known to be effective for their tumors. Plus, participants may benefit from the treatment being evaluated, as in the case of the levamisole + fluorouracil testing.

Clinical trials must be distinguished, however, from what are generously called "unconventional" or "alternative" cancer treatments, less kindly referred to as "quackery." These treatments lie outside of the mainstream of medical practice and have not passed the scrutiny of rigorous animal testing and clinical trial to establish their validity. In the end, the only way to determine whether a treatment works is to compare patients who have received the treatment in question with those who have not. This is the outcome of a phase III clinical trial, which is undertaken only on the basis of positive results in animals as well as in phase I and II trials in humans. Only if patients receiving the treatment in a phase III trial respond favorably compared to controls is the treatment considered beneficial. "Unconventional" cancer treatments do not undergo such objective evaluation but are offered to the public on the basis of limited experience that is not broadly accepted in science or medicine.

Laetrile, a naturally occurring substance extracted from the pits of apricots and other fruits, is a good example of such an unconventional cancer treatment. Laetrile was first used to treat cancer in the 1950s and became popular in the 1970s, when several members of the John Birch Society founded the Committee for the Freedom of Choice in Cancer Therapy, the goal of which was to promote the right of cancer patients to use laetrile. Approximately 70,000 people used laetrile as an anticancer drug during this period, in spite of the fact that a variety of studies in experimental animals failed to detect any antitumor activity. Nonetheless, because of its prominence as an unconventional treatment, the National Cancer Institute undertook phase I and II trials of laetrile. These clinical trials, completed in the early 1980s, again failed to support any claims for laetrile's antitumor activity.

Laetrile, like other unconventional treatments, thus failed to meet objective criteria for activity as an anticancer drug. Nonetheless, it is still offered to the public in Mexican clinics as an effective treatment. There are multiple dangers to cancer patients who go the route of such unconventional therapies. Not only may they be denying themselves the potential benefits of established therapies, but the unconventional treatments may be dangerous in themselves. Laetrile, for example, breaks down in the body to form cyanide, which has led to toxic effects in many patients. There are many other examples of such dangerous treatments. Their effectiveness is highly touted by their proponents, the lack of objective evidence notwithstanding. It is important for patients and family members to be aware of this problem, and to make sure that any proposed treatment has a recognized scientific and medical basis.

SUMMARY

The limiting factor in cancer treatment is metastasis. Localized cancers can usually be effectively treated by surgery or radiotherapy, but over half of cancers have already metastasized to distant body sites by the time of diagnosis. A variety of chemotherapeutic drugs are then used to attempt to kill cancer cells throughout the body. These drugs are usually administered in combinations, in order to maximize their effects and to eliminate cancer cells that may become resistant to any one of the drugs being used. Unfortunately, the chemotherapeutic drugs currently available are not specific for cancer cells. Rather, they interfere generally with cell division and, therefore, also act against those normal cells in the body that are undergoing active proliferation—particularly the blood-forming cells of the bone marrow, the cells that line the intestine, and the cells that form hair. Toxicity to these normal cell populations limits the doses of chemotherapeutic drugs that can be tolerated by the patient and, therefore, limits the effectiveness of chemotherapy. Thus, while some types of cancer are particularly drug-sensitive and can be successfully treated, many cancers are not responsive to current chemotherapy protocols. In some cases, hormones can be used to inhibit the growth of cancer cells, but these treatments usually slow tumor progression rather than eliminating the cancer altogether. Immunotherapy, the manipulation of the immune system to more effectively fight cancer, is an area of active research that has shown promise as a treatment for some cancers but has not yet achieved broad clinical application. It is clear that significant strides in the treatment of cancer have been made; over 50 percent of cancer patients can now be cured. Treatment of the most common kinds of cancer, however, is ineffective once metastasis has occurred, so nearly half of all cancer patients still die of their disease. The yet unmet challenge in cancer treatment is the development of drugs that act specifically against cancer cells.

Chapter 11

Living with Cancer

The occurrence of cancer is a feared and traumatic event in the lives of both patients and their families. Yet, because it is so common in our society, many of us will have to deal with the disease, either as it affects ourselves or our loved ones. The diagnosis of cancer immediately raises the specter of imminent, painful death—and the fear that nothing can be done. Fortunately, today, this is very seldom the case. Something can almost always be done. Over half of all cancer patients can now be cured. In many other cases, although a cure is not ultimately achieved, life can be prolonged for many years by effective treatments. The diagnosis of cancer is no longer a death sentence, and many people must learn to live with cancer as a chronic disease. This chapter discusses some of the problems commonly faced by cancer patients, and some of the support systems patients and their families have found useful in coping with this disease.

DEALING WITH THE DIAGNOSIS OF CANCER

The diagnosis of cancer is horrifying news. In some cases, the patient may seek the advice of the doctor because of symptoms of which he or she is aware, such as a persistent cough or a lump detected during breast self-examination. In other cases, the first signs of cancer may be detected during a routine physical examination or by one of the cancer screening tests (e.g., mammography) discussed in chapter 9. In either event, the first suspicions of cancer must be evaluated by further tests, usually including a biopsy, before a definitive diagnosis can be reached. Learning that cancer is suspected leaves the patient in a state of acute anxiety and uncertainty, which persists until the tests are concluded. If the test results are positive, the emotional impact of a diagnosis of cancer is shattering. Many patients and family members react with mixtures of disbelief, fear, anger, and despair. Indeed, most people are unable to accept and understand a diagnosis of cancer immediately. It takes time for the information to sink in and for its impact to be absorbed.

Anxiety, depression, and hopelessness are common reactions, experienced by many cancer patients. How each patient can best cope with these emotions is a highly individual matter. Once the diagnosis is shared, the support of family and friends is a major resource for many people. Clergy, nurses, and social workers, in addition to physicians, can also be helpful in facing the impact of cancer. Many hospitals offer group as well as individual counseling for cancer patients. In addition, many patients and their families benefit from participation in community support groups. Many such cancer-patient support groups are local chapters of national organizations such as the American Cancer Society. The appendix provides addresses and further information on a number of support groups for cancer patients and their families.

The diagnosis of cancer in a child is particularly devastating to parents and family. Parents must deal with their own feelings of anger, helplessness, and often, guilt. In addition, they must face multiple problems in dealing not only with the sick child, but also with his or her siblings. Assistance in coping with these issues may be sought from a number of support groups, such as the Candlelighters Childhood Cancer Foundation, that are specifically committed to helping families of childhood cancer patients.

One frequent reaction to the diagnosis of cancer is to seek a second opinion. This is usually both wise and appropriate, not just to be sure that the initial diagnosis is correct, but because of the gravity of both the disease and the likely treatments, such as surgery or chemotherapy. It is only prudent to be sure that one is proceeding on the basis of the best possible advice. In many cases, cancer will have been diagnosed by the patient's general physician and it then only makes sense to consult a cancer specialist, called an oncologist. It is important to remember that no doctor should be offended by a patient wishing a second opinion and that the doctor is there to serve the patient. Consultation with a second physician is not only legitimate but may often be valuable to the primary physician as well as to the patient. Indeed, it is usually useful to involve the primary physician in the choice of a consultant, thereby establishing an atmosphere of cooperation—a team effort working for the benefit of the patient. Local cancer specialists may be found by calling the Cancer Information Service of the National Cancer Institute (1–800–4–CANCER) or at Comprehensive Cancer Centers (see appendix).

CANCER TREATMENTS AND THEIR SIDE EFFECTS

Following the diagnosis of cancer, the patient is faced with the necessity of treatments that may seem as devastating as the disease itself. It is particularly critical to select the optimal type of initial treatment, because this is the stage at which a cure is most likely to be achieved. Cancers that recur after the initial therapy is complete have usually progressed to still more malignant diseases, and a complete cure is less likely. Therefore, consultation with an oncologist can be extremely important in deciding on the initial treatment strategy. The optimal treatment program for each patient will depend, not only on the type of cancer, but also on the clinical stage and other characteristics of the particular tumor. The patient's general state of health and other medical conditions also contribute to choices among treatment options. Consequently, it is not unusual for different patients with the same type of cancer to be treated differently.

It is important to remember that, although all cancers have many fundamental properties in common, each cancer is, to some extent, a unique entity. Therefore, the patient's most common questions—What are my chances? or How long do I have?—are often difficult to answer with any precision. For some cancers, the situation is clearcut; the likelihood of a cure is either very high or very low. In many cases, however, current treatments are curative for some, but not all, patients with a particular stage tumor. For example, approximately half of patients with colon cancer which has spread to regional lymph nodes are cured of their disease. Statistics of this type provide an estimate of each patient's chances, but they clearly do not define the outcome for any given individual. Each patient will either be cured or not—an outcome of 100 percent for that person—and survival times can vary substantially from one patient to another. Consequently, each patient must cope, step by step, with his or her individual disease. As noted above, cancer patient support groups can be valuable sources of both information and emotional support for the patient as well as family members.

As discussed in chapter 10, surgery is the initial treatment for many cancers, and it may also play a role in advanced cancer management. For some cancers, surgical removal results in disfigurement or disablement. Examples include amputation of a limb for bone cancer, removal of a breast, loss of speech from removal of the vocal cords (laryngectomy), radical surgery for head and neck cancers, impotence resulting from surgery for prostate cancer, and loss of bowel or bladder control as a result of surgery for intestinal or bladder cancers. In many cases, less radical surgical treatments, often in combination with radiation and/or chemotherapy, can be used. For example, depending on the stage of disease, breast cancer today is often treated by limited surgery rather than mastectomy, and laryngeal cancer may be treated by radiation instead of surgery.

When radical surgery is required, patients may be assisted in dealing with the side effects in a number of ways. For women who have undergone mastectomy, a variety of breast prostheses are available, and breast reconstruction is also a possible option. The Reach to Recovery program of the American Cancer Society (see appendix) is specifically designed to help women who have had mastectomies.

Most patients who have undergone laryngectomy learn to speak again, either using esophageal speech or other methods, with the help of a speech therapist. The International Association of Laryngectomees, which is affiliated with the American Cancer Society, is specifically devoted to providing support for these patients.

An ostomy is a surgical procedure that creates a new opening to the surface of the body. The most common such operation is colostomy, which may be necessary to remove tumors in the lower part of the rectum. The remaining part of the colon is then brought through the wall of the abdomen, and bowel movements are received in a pouch worn over the opening. Ileostomy is a similar operation for cancer of the small intestine. A urostomy may be required for treatment of bladder cancer, in which case urine is collected in a pouch worn over an opening near the navel. These can be lifesaving surgeries, but dealing with an ostomy is clearly a major adjustment. The United Ostomy Association is an organization of over 50,000 people who have had ostomies, and is specifically devoted to helping others cope with these operations.

Radiation treatment and chemotherapy also have serious side effects. Although they are usually reversible, they can be severe during the course of treatment, which commonly lasts for weeks or months. Fatigue is common, resulting from a variety of causes, sometimes including anemia. Nausea, vomiting, and diarrhea are also common side effects, resulting from the action of radiation or chemotherapeutic drugs on the cells that line the intestine. Fortunately, a number of medications to control nausea are now available, and many patients can be helped by these drugs, called antiemetics. The linings of the mouth and throat are also susceptible to radiation and chemotherapeutic drugs, and sore mouths and throats frequently develop as side effects of these treatments. Loss of appetite is a common problem, and it is particularly important for cancer patients to maintain good nutrition in order to prevent weight loss and debilitation. Every effort should be made to make eating as enjoyable as possible, and changes in food preparation and eating practices may be helpful. In some cases, special dietary plans or medication may be needed in this regard. Patients are also frequently susceptible to infections as a result of immune suppression from chemotherapeutic drugs. It is important for patients to avoid possible sources of infection as much as possible, and to seek prompt treatment should signs of infection become evident. Finally, hair loss is a common side effect of cancer chemotherapy. Although temporary, this can have a marked effect on the patient's self-image. The American Cancer Society has developed a support program, called Look Good...Feel Better, which is specifically designed to teach women cosmetic skills to help cope with such treatment side effects.

CANCER AND SEXUALITY

Sexual difficulties, arising from a variety of causes, are experienced by many cancer patients. For patients with cancers of the reproductive organs, such as the penis or vagina, sexual function may be impaired as a direct result of surgical treatment. In other cases, the normal sexual activity of cancer patients may be compromised as a result of stress, disfiguring treatments, or an irrational fear that their cancer is contagious.

For women, surgical treatment of some cancers of the uterine cervix, as well as vaginal cancers, may require removal of the vagina, with obviously drastic effects on sexual function. Some women may cease sexual activity altogether, others may continue to enjoy noncoital sexual relations, and others may choose to have reconstructive surgery of the vagina. Surgical treatment of cancer of the vulva (the external female genitals) has similarly severe effects, compounded by feelings of mutilation. Sexual intercourse remains possible, however, since the vagina is still intact. Finally, women who have undergone radiation treatment for cervical cancer, or hysterectomy for uterine or ovarian cancer, may experience difficulty in intercourse due to vaginal dryness. This can be relieved by the use of lubricants.

Surgical treatment for cancer of the penis has obviously severe consequences for men. If only part of the penis is removed, it is still possible to attain erection and have intercourse. Even if the entire penis is removed, other forms of sexual activity are still possible and orgasms may still be experienced. In addition, there are several kinds of prosthetic devices that can be inserted in the penis to make intercourse possible. Testicular cancers are frequently treated by removal of the affected testicle, but removal of a single testicle impairs neither potency nor fertility. Surgical treatment of prostate cancer used to result in nerve damage leading to impotence for almost all patients, but improved surgical techniques now result in the recovery of potency in many cases. Radiation therapy is an alternative treatment for localized prostate cancer; it usually does not impair potency. However, advanced prostate cancer patients may suffer impotence as a result of hormone treatments.

In addition to these direct effects of cancer on sexual activity, other factors also frequently impair the normal sexual enjoyment of cancer patients. The stress, anxiety, and depression felt by cancer patients and their partners take a natural toll on sexual relations. Patience and communication between partners are critical, and counseling by a sex therapist may be beneficial. One major problem can be the patient's self-image after disfiguring surgery. Because of its sexual significance, removal of a breast is a particularly poignant example. Ostomy patients also frequently experience difficulties for this reason.

One misplaced fear which sometimes impairs sexuality is the notion that cancer is contagious. With the exception of some of the virus-associated cancers discussed in chapter 5, such as anogenital cancers induced by papillomaviruses and cancers associated with AIDS, this is simply not the case. Most cancers are *not* contagious, and unrealistic fears of catching the disease by contact (sexual or otherwise) with a cancer patient can and should be put aside.

INSURANCE AND EMPLOYMENT

Cancer patients and their families often must deal with financial, as well as medical, problems. Cancer is a costly disease, and high treatment costs are frequently compounded by loss of employment income. Furthermore, obtaining insurance coverage and returning to work after treatment can also present special difficulties for cancer survivors.

Health insurance frequently covers some, but not all, of the expenses associated with cancer treatment. Extents of coverage and particular costs that are allowed can vary substantially among different policies. Handling insurance claims and attempting to deal with disallowed costs can be an exceedingly frustrating experience, particularly for a patient undergoing cancer therapy. Hospital business offices or social service departments can be helpful in dealing with insurance companies to resolve any problems.

Although existing insurance policies generally remain in effect, their costs and benefits may change following treatment for cancer. Moreover, obtaining new health and life insurance policies, as may be required for individuals who change jobs, is generally a problem for patients who have been treated for cancer. It should be noted that some states sell health insurance to residents who are unable to find private insurance due to serious medical conditions. State insurance departments will also deal with complaints filed by individuals who feel that they have been unfairly treated by private insurance companies.

Employment is not only a source of income but also an integral part of normal life for many people. Returning to work after treatment, however, can be a major problem for cancer patients. In some cases, disability may make it impossible to return to one's previous job. In other cases, employers and coworkers may be uncomfortable with or discriminate against cancer patients. Reluctance to hire a person who has had cancer may make it difficult to change jobs or find new employment, a difficulty that can be compounded by problems in obtaining the new insurance coverage associated with a job change. It is estimated that about 25 percent of cancer survivors encounter some form of employment discrimination. Help in dealing with these problems may be obtained from a variety of sources, including the American Cancer Society and the National Coalition for Cancer Survivorship (see appendix). It may also be useful to note that employment discrimination against cancer patients was made illegal by the Federal Rehabilitation Act of 1973, which applies to federal employers and all companies receiving federal funding.

SURVIVING CANCER: WILL IT COME BACK?

For many cancer patients, completion of the initial treatment is the beginning of a long period of uncertainty. Was the cancer successfully eliminated, or will it recur? Recurrent cancer may arise either from cells in the vicinity of the primary tumor or from cells that have metastasized to other body sites, most frequently the lungs, liver, bones, or brain. The possibility of recurrent or metastatic cancer is a source of continual anxiety, since only time will tell whether the initial treatment was successful in eliminating all of the cancer cells. Patients must return to their doctors for regular testing, as well as remain alert to possible signs of recurrence of their disease. Although the likelihood of recurrence diminishes with time, it remains an ominous possibility for years after completion of initial treatment.

If cancer does recur, the patient is faced with the fact that a cure is now relatively unlikely. However, many treatments are still available, both to control the cancer and to provide relief from pain and other symptoms of the disease. Treatment of metastatic cancer depends on both the type of cancer and the sites of metastasis. Isolated metastatic tumors in sites such as the liver or lungs may be removed surgically, and radiation or chemotherapy may also be used to slow tumor growth and relieve pain. Advanced prostate cancer, for example, can be treated by hormone therapy which, although not curative, slows tumor growth, relieves pain, and prolongs the lives of many patients. Although some patients with recurrent cancer can still be cured, many are now faced with coping with an incurable chronic disease. Help with some of the associated emotional problems, both for patients and their families, may be sought from both support groups and mental health professionals.

CANCER PAIN

Many people associate cancer with an inevitable, painful death, so cancer pain is frequently a dominant concern for both patients and their families. Unquestionably, pain is a major problem for patients with advanced cancer. However, it is also true that much can be done to control cancer pain, and treatments are now available that provide satisfactory management of pain for the majority of patients.

Pain is seldom a problem in early stages of disease but does affect the majority of patients with advanced cancer. In many cases, pain is not severe and can be controlled with common pain relievers, such as aspirin or Tylenol. Other patients suffer more severe pain, but a variety of effective therapies are available to provide relief. Medications run the gamut from drugs like aspirin, to weak narcotics (e.g., codeine), to strong narcotics (e.g., morphine). Appropriate use of these drugs is successful in relieving pain for most patients, and such pain therapy is an important part of the management of advanced cancer. Indeed, in the terminal stages of disease, relief of pain is the most important service the physician can provide.

It is important for patients to recognize that medications for pain relief should be taken on a regular schedule in order to prevent pain, rather than just being used when pain becomes severe. Moreover, patients and their families should not resist the use of narcotics, such as morphine, for pain relief. Drug tolerance and addiction are not problems under these circumstances, and the stigma attached to recreational use of narcotics does not apply to their use by cancer patients under the care of a physician.

TERMINAL CANCER

In spite of advances in treatment, nearly half of all cancer patients eventually die of their disease. Cancer can kill by invading and interfering with the function of vital organs or by causing other complications, such as hemorrhage or blockage of blood vessels. However, the major single cause of death for cancer patients is infection. In the terminal stages of illness, cancer patients become susceptible to infection due to the debilitating effects of both the cancer and its treatment. Normal body defenses are compromised, and patients often develop and succumb to infections that would not be a problem for healthy individuals.

When there is no longer any expectation of improvement, the goals of treatment become comfort and relief from pain. The patient and family members may wish to consider whether they would want life to be prolonged by extraordinary medical procedures in the event of failure of a vital body function. A document known as a Living Will, obtainable from an organization called Concern for Dying (see appendix), may be used to state the patient's desire for a natural death should this be the case.

Terminal patients (and their families) may also wish to consider whether they would prefer dying at home rather than in the hospital. Families who would rather provide home care can be assisted by hospices, which are specifically designed to provide care and support for terminally ill patients and their families in the home. The general goal of the hospice program is to allow patients to live their last days with their families in as much comfort as possible. Further information may be obtained from the National Hospice Organization (see appendix).

SUMMARY

Cancer patients face an array of physical and emotional problems. The diagnosis of cancer is devastating news, in spite of the fact that effective treatments for most cancers are now available. It is important to remember that over half of cancer patients are cured of their disease and, even if a cure is not achieved, appropriate therapy usually both prolongs and enhances the quality of life. However, the complications of cancer treatment may be severe, sometimes including disabling or disfiguring surgery. Common side effects of radiation and chemotherapy include fatigue, nausea, vomiting, diarrhea, sore mouths and throats, loss of appetite, susceptibility to infections, and hair loss. Sexual difficulties are also experienced by many cancer patients. These medical problems are frequently compounded by difficulties with insurance coverage and employment. These problems are commonly experienced by cancer patients, and a variety of support groups (see appendix) are available to help patients and their families.

For patients with advanced cancer, dealing with pain becomes a major concern. Fortunately, current treatments are able to provide effective pain relief for the majority of patients. Terminally ill patients and their families may wish to consider hospice programs designed to provide home care and pain relief, thereby enabling patients to spend their last days at home with their families.

PART IV

Overview of Major Types of Cancer

Chapter 12

Leukemias and Lymphomas

Leukemias and lymphomas are cancers of the blood and lymph systems. Together, they account for approximately 8 percent of United States cancer incidence, or about 82,000 cases annually. In addition, leukemias and lymphomas are the most common cancers in children, representing about half of all childhood malignancies, or approximately 3,800 cases annually.

There are many different types of leukemias and lymphomas, depending on the type of cell involved and how rapidly the disease progresses. All of the different cells in blood and lymph are derived from a common precursor cell, called the pluripotent stem cell, in bone marrow. Leukemias and lymphomas result from the continuous proliferation of cells that are blocked at various stages of their normal differentiation to specialized cell types (Fig. 12.1). The first step in blood-cell differentiation gives rise to myeloid and lymphoid progenitor cells. Cells derived from the myeloid lineage include blood platelets, red blood cells, granulocytes, monocytes, and macrophages. These cells function in blood coagulation (platelets), oxygen transport (red blood cells), inflammatory reactions (granulocytes, monocytes, and macrophages), and the immune response (macrophages). The lymphoid lineage gives rise to B and T lymphocytes, which are responsible for antibody secretion and cell-mediated immunity, respectively. B lymphocytes develop within the bone marrow, whereas the precursors of T lymphocytes migrate to the thymus and develop there. Precursors of both B and T lymphocytes then migrate to the lymphatic system, which includes the lymph nodes and spleen plus the thymus, tonsils, adenoids, and aggregates of lymphatic tissue in the bone marrow and intestine (Fig. 12.2). In addition to lymphocytes, lymphatic tissues contain macrophages; both function in the immune response.

Leukemias arise in the blood-forming cells of the bone marrow, and can result from abnormal proliferation of any of the different kinds of cells within either the myeloid or lymphoid lineages. Lymphomas, by contrast, develop from lymphocytes or macrophages in lymphatic

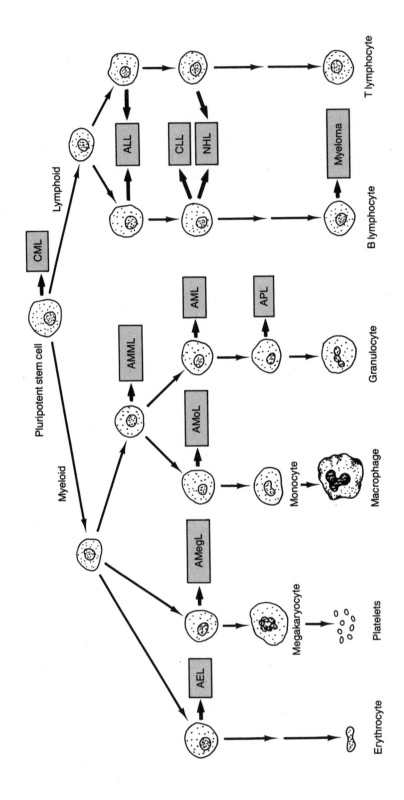

Table 12.1
THE MOST COMMON LEUKEMIAS AND LYMPHOMAS

Type of Cancer	Approximate Cases per Year (United States population)	
	Children	Adults
Acute lymphocytic leukemia	1,900	3,000
Acute nonlymphocytic leukemia	600	8,000
Chronic lymphocytic leukemia	—	8,000
Chronic myelogenous leukemia	100	5,000
Hodgkin's disease	500	7,000
Non-Hodgkin's lymphomas	700	35,000
Multiple myeloma	—	12,000
Total	3,800	78,000

tissues. In children, leukemias are about twice as frequent as lymphomas, whereas lymphomas are more common in adults. The most prevalent of these diseases (Table 12.1) are discussed in this chapter.

ACUTE LYMPHOCYTIC LEUKEMIA

Acute lymphocytic leukemia (ALL) is the most common leukemia in children, accounting for approximately 1900 cases of childhood leukemia annually in the United States (approximately 75% of childhood leukemias and 25% of all cancers in children). It is less common in adults,

← Figure 12.1

Cellular origins of leukemias and lymphomas. Different kinds of leukemias and lymphomas most frequently result from continued proliferation of cells blocked at the indicated stages of their normal differentiation. CML is chronic myelogenous leukemia; AEL, acute erythroid leukemia; AMegL, acute megakaryocytic leukemia; AMoL, acute monocytic leukemia; AMML, acute myelomonocytic leukemia; AML, acute myelocytic leukemia; APL, acute promyelocytic leukemia; ALL, acute lymphocytic leukemia; CLL, chronic lymphocytic leukemia; and NHL, non-Hodgkin's lymphomas.

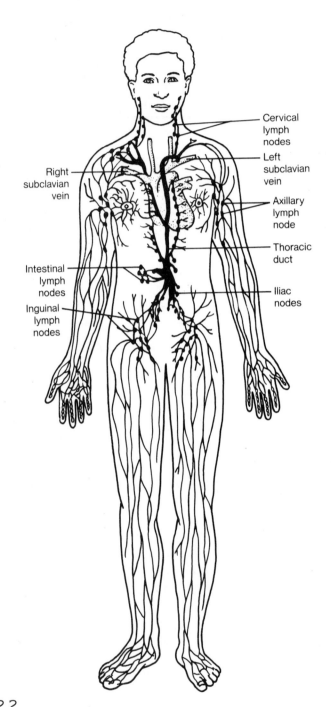

Cervical
lymph
nodes

Left
subclavian
vein

Right
subclavian
vein

Axillary
lymph
node

Thoracic
duct

Intestinal
lymph
nodes

Iliac
nodes

Inguinal
lymph
nodes

Figure 12.2

The lymphatic system.

where it represents about 12 percent of all leukemias. Acute lymphocytic leukemia is a rapidly progressing, or acute, disease characterized by an abnormal increase in immature lymphocytes (lymphocytic) in the blood and bone marrow (Fig. 12.1). About 20 percent of these leukemias arise from T cells, the remainder being of B-cell origin.

The causes of most cases of ALL (and other leukemias) are unknown, although the risk of ALL is increased by exposure to radiation. In addition, ALL occurs more frequently in individuals with some inherited diseases that are associated with instability of the genetic material, including Down's syndrome, Fanconi's anemia, Bloom's syndrome, and ataxia telangiectasia (see chapter 6). Consistent with this general association of DNA damage with increased leukemia risk, a number of alterations in oncogenes and tumor suppressor genes are frequently observed in ALL.

Early detection of ALL, like other leukemias, is difficult. Initial symptoms are usually nonspecific, resembling those associated with common infectious diseases, such as fever and fatigue. Additional signs of disease include frequent infections, a tendency to bleed or bruise easily, paleness, and weight loss. When leukemia is suspected, diagnosis is made by microscopic examination of the blood and bone marrow.

Fortunately, ALL, particularly in children, is one of the cancers that responds well to chemotherapy. Indeed, childhood ALL was the first leukemia to be successfully treated with chemotherapy, and has served as a model for the development of current concepts of cancer treatment. The disease is now treated using combinations of drugs, including vincristine, prednisone, asparaginase, doxorubicin, methotrexate, and mercaptopurine. Such combination chemotherapy is curative for more than half of children with this disease. It should be noted, however, that treatment of ALL, like all cancers, is a complicated undertaking, which is best performed by specialized teams with appropriate training and experience. The effectiveness of therapy for childhood ALL indeed varies between different institutions, with cure rates as high as 75 percent in some medical centers. Adult patients with ALL generally respond less well than children, but chemotherapy is still an effective treatment.

ACUTE NONLYMPHOCYTIC LEUKEMIAS

The acute nonlymphocytic leukemias affect blood-cell types other than lymphocytes (Fig. 12.1). The most common is acute myelocytic leukemia (AML), which accounts for the majority of acute leukemias in adults. Other types of acute nonlymphocytic leukemias include acute promyelocytic leukemia, acute myelomonocytic leukemia, acute mono-cytic leukemia, and erythroleukemia. Risk factors and symptoms for these diseases are similar to those discussed for ALL above. Exposure to some occupational carcinogens, such as benzene (see chapter 4), also increases the risk of AML. In addition, some of the drugs used in cancer chemotherapy, particularly the alkylating agents which induce DNA damage (see chapter 10), can lead to the development of secondary leukemias. *Ras* oncogenes are frequently involved in AML, often playing a role early in the disease process. Interestingly, acute promyelocytic leukemia is characterized by mutations converting the retinoic acid receptor gene to an oncogene, which appears to contribute to the development of this leukemia by preventing normal cell differentiation.

The acute nonlymphocytic leukemias are treated by chemotherapy with combinations of drugs, frequently including daunomycin and cytosine arabinoside. Chemotherapy for the acute nonlymphocytic leukemias is less successful than that for ALL, however, and treatment of the majority of these patients fails to completely eliminate the leukemic cells. The currently used combination chemotherapy protocols are, therefore, curative for only about 20 percent of AML patients. Given the role of the retinoic acid receptor as an oncogene in acute promyelocytic leukemia, it is noteworthy that retinoic acid appears to be of therapeutic benefit in this disease, by inducing differentiation, and thus inhibiting proliferation, of the leukemic cells.

CHRONIC LYMPHOCYTIC LEUKEMIA

Chronic lymphocytic leukemia (CLL) is rare in children but accounts for about one-third of all leukemias in adults. It occurs most frequently in patients over 60 years of age. Usually the leukemic cells are immature B lymphocytes.

CLL is a much more slowly progressing disease than ALL. In the early stages, which may last for many years, patients have no symptoms of disease, and diagnosis is only made by the observation of abnormal numbers of blood lymphocytes. The average survival time is nearly ten years from diagnosis at this stage. Because of its indolent course, treatment of CLL is generally not initiated until symptoms appear. Once symptoms do become evident, patients are treated with low-dose chemotherapy, usually with alkylating agents. Such treatment is not curative, but is usually effective in slowing the course of disease. Because normal function of the immune system is gradually lost as the disease progresses, most patients with CLL die of infection or other illnesses not directly related to the leukemia.

CHRONIC MYELOGENOUS LEUKEMIA

Chronic myelogenous leukemia (CML) is also a slowly progressing disease, which is rare in children but accounts for approximately 20 percent of adult leukemias. It originates in the pluripotent stem cell in the bone marrow—the cell that gives rise to all the different cell types of the hematopoietic system, including cells of both the lymphoid and myeloid lineages (see Fig. 12.1). It is characterized predominantly by the accumulation of abnormal numbers of granulocytes in the blood and bone marrow. As discussed in chapter 9, CML always involves activation of the *abl* oncogene by rearrangement of DNA from chromosome 9 to chromosome 22, a chromosomal rearrangement known as the Philadelphia translocation, after the city in which it was discovered. Because this oncogene translocation is universally present in the leukemic cells, it is an important diagnostic marker for following the status of disease in CML patients.

The course of CML is divided into two stages: chronic phase and blast crisis. The chronic phase of the disease is associated with minimal symptoms and may persist for years. Eventually, however, patients progress to an accelerated stage of the disease, which culminates in the acute, life-threatening phase known as blast crisis. Blast crisis resembles an acute leukemia and is characterized by the accumulation of large numbers of rapidly proliferating leukemic cells, called blasts. The blast cells are myeloid in about two-thirds of cases, and lymphoid in the remainder. One of the events involved in progression from the chronic phase of CML to blast crisis may be mutation of the *p53* tumor suppressor gene.

CML patients in blast crisis are treated with chemotherapy regimens similar to those used in ALL or AML, depending on whether the blast cells are lymphoid or myeloid. If successful, such therapy may induce remission to the chronic phase. Chemotherapy is also used during the chronic phase of the disease, but does not usually succeed in totally eradicating the leukemic cells. Bone marrow transplantation may be curative for up to 50 percent of chronic-phase CML patients, although this procedure is associated with significant risks due to its severely toxic side effects. Treatment risks are lower for patients early in the course of disease, and the cure rate from bone marrow transplantation may be as high as 80 percent if performed within the first year of diagnosis.

HODGKIN'S DISEASE

Hodgkin's disease is the most frequent type of lymphoma, accounting for about 7400 cases annually in the United States. It frequently affects young adults, with most cases occurring between the ages of 15 and 35. No known causes or risk factors for Hodgkin's disease have been identified, in spite of some speculation that it may be associated with an infectious agent.

The site of origin of Hodgkin's disease is a lymph node, frequently in the neck. It then spreads through the lymph system and, in advanced stages, affects other organs, including the spleen, liver, lungs, and bone marrow. The initial symptom is usually painless lymph-node enlargement, sometimes accompanied by fever, night sweats, itching of the skin, or weight loss. Diagnosis is made by microscopic examination of a lymph node biopsy.

Hodgkin's disease is distinguished by the presence of a unique type of cell, called the Reed-Sternberg cell, in affected lymph nodes. Unlike most cancers, the bulk of the tumor mass in Hodgkin's disease is composed of normal lymphocytes and connective tissue, rather than of tumor cells. The Reed-Sternberg cell, which is probably of lymphoid origin, appears to be the actual malignant cell in the disease.

Hodgkin's disease can be successfully treated by both radiation and chemotherapy. Early stages of the disease, in which only one lymph node is involved or in which only limited spread of the tumor to regional lymph nodes has occurred, can be cured by intensive radiotherapy in nearly 90 percent of cases. Chemotherapy is also effective for both early and advanced stages of Hodgkin's disease. A number of different drug combinations are employed, one example being the regimen called MOPP, which consists of mechlorethamine, vincristine (Oncovin), procarbazine, and prednisone. Such combination chemotherapy is curative for over half of patients with even advanced stages of Hodgkin's disease. Indeed, treatment of Hodgkin's disease has become sufficiently successful that long-term side effects are important concerns, particularly since the disease frequently affects young people. Such treatment side effects include sterility and an increased incidence of secondary leukemias induced by the chemotherapeutic drugs.

NON-HODGKIN'S LYMPHOMAS

Lymphomas other than Hodgkin's disease comprise about 36,000 cases per year in the United States. The majority (about 80%) of non-Hodgkin's lymphomas are malignancies of B lymphocytes, although about 15 percent arise from T lymphocytes and the remaining 5 percent from macrophages. Several kinds of lymphomas, which differ considerably in their causes, prognosis, and treatment, are grouped together under this classification.

A number of different systems have been used to classify the non-Hodgkin's lymphomas according to the type of malignant cell involved and the aggressiveness of the disease. In fact, six different systems are used throughout the world and, in spite of attempts to achieve a uniform classification, no single system has yet been broadly accepted. One of the most commonly used classifications is the Rappaport system (Table 12.2). In this scheme, lymphomas are first classified by growth pattern, either nodular or diffuse. They are then subclassified by cell type: lymphocytic if the cells are small and resemble lymphocytes; histiocytic if the cells are large and resemble macrophages or histiocytes; and mixed if the cells are of both sizes. Finally, the lymphoma cells are further described as well differentiated or poorly differentiated, depending on their extent of morphological similarity to normal cells. This system is unsatisfactory principally because the classification of cell types is a description of morphology that does not correctly identify the actual origin of the malignant cell. In particular, the so called histiocytic lymphomas are most frequently malignancies of B lymphocytes, not of histiocytes (macrophages). Nonetheless, since the Rappaport system correctly

Table 12.2
NON-HODGKIN'S LYMPHOMAS

Rappaport Classification	Type of Cell	Percent of Cases
Low Grade		
Diffuse well-differentiated lymphocytic	B	10–15
Nodular poorly differentiated lymphocytic	B	15–20
Nodular mixed lymphocytic-histiocytic	B	5–10
Intermediate Grade		
Nodular histiocytic	B	<5
Diffuse poorly differentiated lymphocytic	B or T	15–20
Diffuse mixed lymphocytic-histiocytic	B or T	5–10
Diffuse histiocytic	B or T	30
High Grade		
Diffuse histiocytic	B or T	5–10
Diffuse lymphoblastic	T	<5
Diffuse undifferentiated	B	<5

predicts biological behavior and clinical response, it remains one of the most widely used classifications of lymphomas and will, therefore, form the basis of the present discussion.

Several types of lymphomas—the intermediate and high-grade classes—are aggressive malignancies which grow rapidly and are quickly fatal if not treated. These include nodular and diffuse histiocytic lymphoma, diffuse lymphoblastic lymphoma, diffuse poorly differentiated lymphocytic lymphoma, diffuse undifferentiated lymphoma, and diffuse mixed lymphocytic-histiocytic lymphoma. About half of patients with non-Hodgkin's lymphomas have one of these aggressive diseases, and they are the most common lymphomas in children.

Other lymphomas, the low-grade ones, are referred to as indolent diseases because, like the chronic leukemias, they grow slowly and may persist for years with minimal symptoms. These tumors, which usually occur in adults, include nodular poorly differentiated lymphocytic lymphoma, diffuse well-differentiated lymphocytic lymphoma, and nodular mixed lymphocytic-histiocytic lymphoma. In time, however, these indolent lymphomas evolve to more aggressive diseases, accompanied by symptoms such as fever, night sweats, and weight loss.

Epstein-Barr virus (EBV) is a causative agent of Burkitt's lymphoma, a diffuse undifferentiated lymphoma in the Rappaport system, which occurs with a high incidence in some regions of Africa (see chapter 5). In addition, EBV is associated with the high frequency of lymphomas in immune deficient patients. As discussed in chapters 4, 5, and 6, patients with inherited or acquired immunodeficiencies (resulting from immunosuppressive drugs or AIDS) develop EBV-associated B-cell lymphomas about a hundred times more frequently than the general population.

Burkitt's and other aggressive B-cell lymphomas regularly involve the c-*myc* oncogene, as discussed in chapter 7. In contrast, the indolent follicular (nodular) B-cell lymphomas involve a different oncogene, *bcl*-2. The *bcl*-2 oncogene is unusual in that it acts to prolong cell survival rather than promote active cell proliferation—an activity that seems consistent with the slow progression of these indolent diseases. The progression of indolent lymphomas to more aggressive growth may involve activation of c-*myc* as a second event, resulting in increased tumor cell proliferation.

The prognosis for patients with lymphomas seems paradoxical, in that the more aggressive lymphomas are more curable than are the indolent ones. In particular, the aggressive lymphomas respond well to combination chemotherapy, which is curative in over 50 percent of cases. Commonly used drugs include cyclophosphamide, vincristine, procarbazine, and prednisone. The indolent lymphomas are also treated by chemotherapy and radiation, but not usually cured. In many cases, symptom-free patients with indolent lymphomas are closely monitored but do not receive treatment unless the disease shows signs of progressing to a more aggressive form.

MULTIPLE MYELOMA

Multiple myeloma is a neoplasm of plasma cells, which are mature antibody-secreting B lymphocytes. There are about 12,000 cases annually in the United States. Multiple myeloma usually develops in older adults, with the average age of onset being around 70. Initial symptoms usually include bone pain, anemia, and fatigue. In addition to microscopic examination of blood and bone marrow, diagnosis includes analysis of blood and urine for antibodies secreted by the myeloma cells. There are no established causes or reproducible genetic alterations associated with multiple myeloma in humans, although the c-*myc* oncogene is involved in a closely related cancer (plasmacytoma) in mice. The disease is usually treated by chemotherapy, with combinations of drugs including alkylating agents (melphalan or cyclophosphamide) and prednisone. Such treatment is frequently effective in controlling disease progression for a period of two to four years, but is not generally curative.

SUMMARY

Leukemias and lymphomas are cancers of the blood and lymph systems. They comprise about half of all childhood cancers, and about 8 percent of cancers in adults. In most cases, the causes are unknown, although infection with Epstein-Barr virus in combination with immunodeficiency results in a high risk of lymphoma development. Different types of leukemias and lymphomas involve several oncogenes and tumor suppressor genes, some of which affect cell differentiation and cell survival, as well as cell proliferation. Leukemias are treated by chemotherapy; and lymphomas by both chemotherapy and radiation. Such treatments are effective for several of the most virulent of these diseases, including acute lymphocytic leukemia—the most common childhood cancer—Hodgkin's disease, and aggressive non-Hodgkin's lymphomas.

Chapter 13

Childhood Solid Tumors

Childhood cancer is rare, accounting for approximately 7600 cases annually in the United States, or less than 1 percent of the total cancer incidence. On the other hand, cancer is second only to accidents as the leading cause of death in children under age 15. The common adult cancers (such as cancers of the lung, breast, colon, and prostate) occur very infrequently in children. Instead, as discussed in the preceding chapter, about half of childhood cancers are leukemias and lymphomas. The remainder are varieties of solid tumors (Table 13.1) that are rare in adults. Many of these tumors are evident soon after birth, and probably arise during early embryonic development. In general, childhood tumors are rapidly growing cancers that are often more responsive to chemotherapy than the common solid tumors of adults.

Table 13.1
CHILDHOOD CANCERS

Type of Cancer	Approximate Cases per Year (United States Population)	
Leukemias and lymphomas	3800	(50%)
Brain tumors	1500	(20%)
Neuroblastoma	600	(8%)
Wilms' tumor	400	(5%)
Bone tumors	400	(5%)
Soft-tissue sarcomas	400	(5%)
Retinoblastoma	200	(3%)
	7300	(96%)

Percentages refer to total estimated incidence of all cancers in children under 15.

BRAIN TUMORS

Brain tumors are the most common solid tumors of childhood, accounting for about 20 percent of all cancers in children. There are several different types of brain tumors, the most common being astrocytomas, medulloblastomas, and ependymomas. Astrocytomas, which account for nearly two-thirds of childhood brain tumors, occur in children of all ages. Ependymomas and medulloblastomas are most frequent in children under age 5 and between the ages of 5 and 10, respectively. The causes and risk factors for the development of childhood brain tumors are not known. In some cases, inactivation of the *p53* tumor suppressor gene may be involved.

Symptoms of brain tumors include headaches, dizziness, blurred vision, and problems with coordination. Diagnosis involves a variety of imaging techniques, particularly CT scan and MRI, as well as recording the brain's electrical activity by electroencephalography (EEG). Surgery is the primary therapy, the goal being to remove the entire tumor. This is not always possible, however, and brain tumors are unusual in that even benign tumors can be life-threatening if their location precludes surgical removal. Tumors that are not accessible to surgery, or that cannot be completely removed, are treated by radiation and chemotherapy, for example, with drugs such as vincristine and actinomycin D.

The overall cure rate for brain tumors in children is greater than 50 percent, but this varies considerably according to the tumor type. Five-year survival rates for children with ependymoma or medulloblastoma are 70 to 80 percent, but the prognosis for children with astrocytomas is less favorable. Low-grade astrocytomas can sometimes be cured by surgery, and five-year survival rates for children with these tumors are around 50 percent, depending on the location of the tumor. The more aggressive astrocytomas—anaplastic astrocytomas and glioblastomas—are more malignant tumors, with average survival times of two to three years and about one year, respectively.

NEUROBLASTOMA

Neuroblastoma is the next most common childhood cancer, accounting for approximately 8 percent of all childhood malignancies. It is a neoplasm of embryonic neural cells that usually occurs by 2 years of age. Rare cases are inherited (see chapter 6), but causes for the majority of cases are unknown. Progression of neuroblastomas to more aggressively growing advanced stages of disease is associated with high levels of expression of the N-*myc* oncogene, as discussed in chapter 7. Once neuroblastomas have progressed to these advanced stages (stages III and IV), they often respond poorly to treatment, so the activity of N-*myc* is an important indicator of prognosis.

Neuroblastomas most frequently originate in the abdomen, and are usually detected as a swelling or abnormal tissue mass. The disease is treated with surgery, radiation, and chemotherapy, using combinations of drugs frequently including cyclophosphamide and doxorubicin. The overall survival rate is about 50 percent, but this is highly dependent on the age of the patient and on the extent of disease progression at the time of diagnosis (Fig. 13.1). In children under 1 year of age, all stages of neuroblastoma can be effectively treated, with cure rates of about 90 percent. In older children, however, only the early stages of disease respond well to therapy. Thus, while 80 to 90 percent of children older than 1 year are cured of stage I and II neuroblastomas, survival rates fall to less than 20 percent for children of these ages having stage III or IV disease.

RETINOBLASTOMA

Retinoblastoma is an eye tumor, arising from embryonic retinal cells, which accounts for about 3 percent of childhood cancers. It usually occurs by age 3. Despite its rarity, retinoblastoma has been important as the prototype example of the involvement of a tumor suppressor gene in inherited cancer (see chapters 6 and 7). Both inherited and noninherited retinoblastomas involve mutations of the *RB* tumor suppressor gene. About 40 percent of retinoblastoma cases are hereditary and arise following inheritance of a defective *RB* gene from one parent. Children with inherited retinoblastoma frequently develop multiple tumors in both eyes.

Retinoblastoma is usually detected by a change in the appearance of the pupil, particularly the occurrence of a white reflection. If diagnosed early, retinoblastoma can be cured by surgery or radiotherapy without loss of vision.

WILMS' TUMOR

Wilms' tumor is a tumor of embryonic kidney cells which accounts for about 5 percent of childhood cancer incidence. It usually occurs by age 5. Like retinoblastoma, Wilms' tumor develops as a result of mutations in a tumor suppressor gene—in this case, a gene called *WT*1. Some cases of Wilms' tumor are inherited, and these are likely to involve the development of multiple tumors in both kidneys. Wilms' tumors are also frequently associated with other congenital abnormalities, including

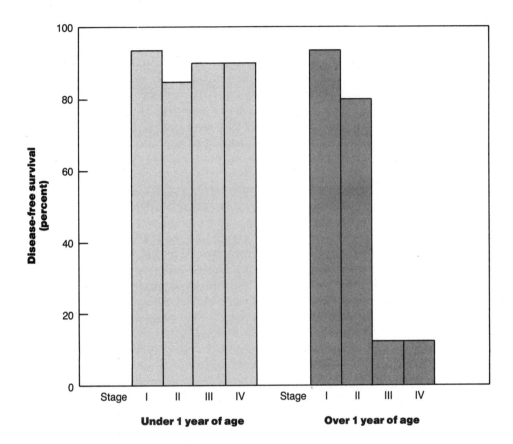

Figure 13.1

Prognosis for children with neuroblastoma. Disease-free survival for children under and over 1 year of age is plotted as a function of the stage of the tumor at diagnosis. The staging system for neuroblastoma is outlined in Table 7.3. (Data from P. A. Pizzo et al. In *Cancer: Principles and Practice of Oncology,* ed. V. T. DeVita, Jr., S. Hellman and S. A. Rosenberg (3rd ed.). Philadelphia: Lippincott, 1989.)

aniridia (absence of the iris), genitourinary defects, and mental retardation (the WAGR syndrome).

Wilms' tumors are usually detected as a swelling or mass in the abdomen, and diagnosed by x-rays and other imaging techniques. Treatment of Wilms' tumor generally involves a combination of surgery, radiation, and chemotherapy, particularly using the drugs actinomycin D and vincristine. The response of Wilms' tumor patients is good, and cures are obtained in over 80 percent of cases.

BONE TUMORS

Two types of bone cancer, osteosarcoma and Ewing's sarcoma, together constitute about 5 percent of childhood malignancies. Both usually occur in children between the ages of 10 and 18. Osteosarcomas involve mutations of the *RB* tumor suppressor gene, and often occur as second tumors in patients with inherited retinoblastoma. The *p53* tumor suppressor gene is also frequently mutated in osteosarcomas.

The primary symptoms of both osteosarcomas and Ewing's sarcomas are pain and swelling in the area of the tumor. Diagnosis is then made by x-rays and biopsy. Both of these bone cancers respond well to treatment. Osteosarcomas are usually treated by surgical removal, coupled with chemotherapy using methotrexate, doxorubicin, and cisplatin. In many cases, it is possible to remove only the section of bone in which the tumor is localized, rather than amputate the entire limb. Ewing's sarcoma is highly sensitive to radiation and is usually treated by radiation plus chemotherapy with drug combinations including vincristine, cyclophosphamide, actinomycin D, and doxorubicin. Cure rates for both these bone cancers are about 50 percent.

SOFT-TISSUE SARCOMAS

Rhabdomyosarcoma, a cancer of skeletal muscle cells, is the most frequent soft-tissue sarcoma in children, accounting for approximately 4 percent of all childhood cancers. It occurs most frequently in children either between the ages of 2 and 6 or 14 and 18. In some cases, rhabdomyosarcomas are inherited, for example, in the Li-Fraumeni cancer family syndrome (see chapter 6). Mutations of the *RB* and *p53* tumor suppressor genes frequently occur in these tumors.

The initial sign of rhabdomyosarcoma is usually a painless lump or mass, which is diagnosed by biopsy. Surgery is the primary treatment, combined with radiation and chemotherapy, depending on the extent of tumor spread. Chemotherapy is effective against rhabdomyosarcoma, usually employing drug combinations that include vincristine, actinomycin D, and cyclophosphamide. The overall survival rate is approximately 70 percent.

Other soft-tissue sarcomas together account for about 1 percent of childhood cancers. They include fibrosarcomas, cancers of fibrous connective tissue; liposarcomas, cancers of fat cells; hemangiopericytomas, cancers of cells that surround the blood vessels; and synovial sarcomas, cancers of cells that line joint cavities and tendon sheaths. The primary treatment for these diseases is surgery, possibly in combination with radiation and chemotherapy.

SUMMARY

Together with the leukemias and lymphomas discussed in chapter 12, the tumors reviewed in this chapter account for about 95 percent of childhood cancers. These tumors occur only rarely in adults, where the vast majority of cancers are solid tumors of other sites. Most cancers of children are rapidly growing malignancies, which frequently arise from embryonal cell types. There are both inherited and noninherited forms of a number of childhood cancers, most notably retinoblastoma and Wilms' tumor. Hereditary cases of these cancers result from inheritance of a defective copy of a tumor suppressor gene, *RB* or *WT1*, respectively. Mutations of the *RB* and *p53* tumor suppressor genes are also important in bone tumors and soft-tissue sarcomas. In addition, the N-*myc* oncogene plays an important role in the progression of neuroblastomas to advanced stages of disease. Many of the childhood cancers are responsive to radiation and chemotherapy, and overall cure rates for these diseases range from 50 to 90 percent.

Chapter 14

Common Solid Tumors of Adults

The majority (about 90%) of adult cancers are carcinomas, that is, cancers arising from the epithelial cells that cover the surface of the body and line the internal organs. Most of the remainder are leukemias and lymphomas, which constitute approximately 8 percent of all adult cancers and were discussed in chapter 12. Sarcomas of bone and soft tissues are very rare in adults, altogether accounting for less than 1 percent of adult cancers. This chapter discusses the common solid tumors of adults in order of their incidence in the United States population (Table 14.1).

LUNG CANCER

Cancer of the lung (Fig. 14.1) is responsible for approximately 15 percent of cancer cases, and 28 percent of cancer deaths, in the United States. As discussed in chapters 4 and 8, 80 to 90 percent of lung cancers are caused by cigarette smoking and, therefore, could be prevented by avoidance of this single carcinogenic agent. Additional risk factors for lung cancer include exposure to excess radon levels in the home and to certain industrial carcinogens such as asbestos. The effect of these carcinogens combines with that of smoking, imparting an extremely high lung cancer risk to smokers exposed to these added carcinogenic insults. As discussed in chapter 6, lung cancer risk may also be affected by inherited differences in sensitivity to carcinogens.

Lung cancers are classified as small-cell and nonsmall-cell carcinomas. The most common nonsmall-cell types are adenocarcinomas, squamous cell carcinomas, and large-cell carcinomas. All types of lung cancer are associated with mutations of the *p53* tumor suppressor gene, and small-cell carcinomas are also associated with mutations of *RB*. In addition, nonsmall-cell carcinomas frequently involve *ras* oncogenes.

Lung cancer is difficult to detect in early stages of the disease process.

Table 14.1
ADULT SOLID TUMORS IN THE UNITED STATES

Type of Cancer	Cases per Year		Deaths per Year	
Lung	157,000	(15%)	142,000	(28%)
Colon/rectum	155,000	(15%)	61,000	(12%)
Breast	151,000	(14%)	44,000	(8.6%)
Prostate	106,000	(10%)	30,000	(5.9%)
Urinary				
Bladder	49,000	(5%)	10,000	(2%)
Kidney	24,000	(2%)	10,000	(2%)
Uterus				
Cervix	13,500	(1%)	6,000	(1.2%)
Endometrium	33,000	(3%)	4,000	(0.8%)
Oral cavity	31,000	(3%)	8,000	(1.6%)
Pancreas	28,000	(3%)	25,000	(5%)
Skin	28,000	(3%)	9,000	(1.8%)
Stomach	23,000	(2%)	14,000	(2.7%)
Ovary	21,000	(2%)	12,000	(2.4%)
Brain	16,000	(1.5%)	11,000	(2.2%)
Liver	15,000	(1.5%)	12,000	(2.4%)
Larynx	12,000	(1%)	4,000	(0.8%)
Thyroid	12,000	(1%)	1,000	(0.2%)
Esophagus	11,000	(1%)	10,000	(2%)
Testis	6,000	(0.6%)	400	(0.1%)
Total	892,000	(84.6%)	413,000	(81.7%)

Percentages refer to total United States cancer incidence and mortality.
Nonmelanoma skin cancers and cervical carcinomas *in situ* are not included in
incidence figures. The remaining cancers not included in this table are the
leukemias and lymphomas (8% of incidence, 9% of mortality), sarcomas (1% of
incidence and mortality), and relatively rare carcinomas of other unspecified
sites. (Data are from American Cancer Society, *Cancer Facts and Figures*, 1990.)

Symptoms, which include persistent cough, chest pain, and sputum
streaked with blood, do not usually appear until the cancer has reached
an advanced stage, at which metastasis has already occurred. Treatment
is usually surgery, combined with radiation and chemotherapy. Lung

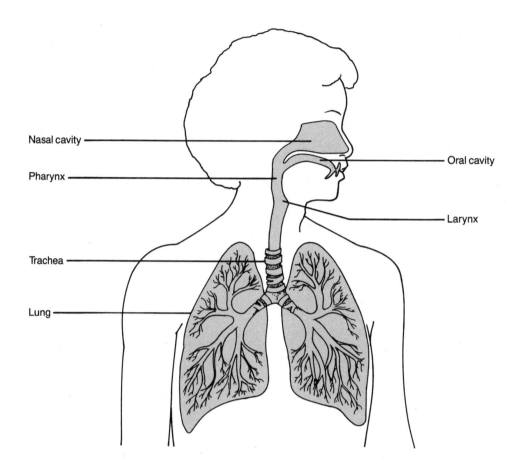

Figure 14.1

The respiratory system.

cancers, however, are not very responsive, and the five-year survival rate is only about 13 percent.

COLON AND RECTUM CANCER

Together, colon and rectum cancers (Fig. 14.2) account for approximately 15 percent of United States cancer incidence and 12 percent of mortality. Cancers of these sites are adenocarcinomas. Colon carcinoma is about twice as common as rectal carcinoma. Rare forms of colon cancer are inherited, for example, familial adenomatous polyposis, as discussed in

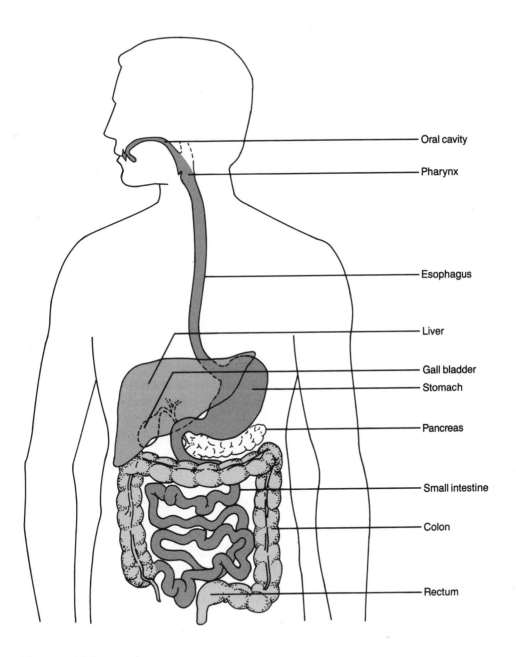

Oral cavity

Pharynx

Esophagus

Liver

Gall bladder

Stomach

Pancreas

Small intestine

Colon

Rectum

Figure 14.2

The digestive system.

chapter 6. In addition, the risk of developing colon and rectum cancers is about twice as high for individuals with an immediate family member who has had the disease as it is for the general population. It has been estimated that increased susceptibility to colon cancer is inherited by 10 to 20 percent of the population, which may contribute to a substantial fraction of cases. Inflammatory bowel disease, for example, ulcerative colitis, is also associated with a high risk of developing colon cancer. An individual who has had one polyp or carcinoma is also at increased risk of developing a second. Dietary factors are thought to be important determinants of the risk of colon and rectum cancers. As discussed in chapters 4 and 8, an increased incidence of these cancers appears to be associated with diets that are high in fat and low in fiber and/or other components of fruits and vegetables. The clearest risk factor is a high-fat (greater than 40 percent of total calories) diet, which appears to result in about a two-fold increase in colon cancer incidence.

Colon and rectum carcinomas are the best characterized cancers with respect to the roles of oncogenes and tumor suppressor genes in tumor development. The *ras*K oncogene and the *APC* and *MCC* tumor suppressor genes appear to be involved in early stages of the disease process, contributing to the development of premalignant adenomas (polyps). Progression to malignant carcinomas then involves loss or inactivation of the *p53* and *DCC* tumor suppressor genes.

In part because of the gradual progression of colon and rectum carcinomas, early detection is a feasible approach to reducing mortality from these cancers. As discussed in chapter 9, early stages of colon and rectum tumors can be detected, albeit with varying degrees of sensitivity and reliability, by digital rectal examination, sigmoidoscopy, and fecal occult blood testing. The use of all three of these screening tests is recommended by the American Cancer Society, particularly after age 50.

The benefits of early detection are apparent in the treatment of colon and rectum cancers, which primarily relies on surgical removal of the tumor, sometimes combined with radiation and chemotherapy. Overall survival is about 50 percent, but this is largely dependent on the extent of tumor progression at the time of diagnosis. Premalignant polyps are readily cured by removal during endoscopy. Cure rates for early-stage localized colon and rectum carcinomas are also high, close to 90 and 80 percent, respectively. After the cancers have spread regionally to lymph nodes and adjacent organs, however, survival rates drop to about 50 percent, and survival rates for patients with distant metastases are less than 10 percent. Postsurgical chemotherapy with fluorouracil + levamisole has recently been found to reduce mortality by about 30 percent for patients with colon cancer that has spread to regional lymph nodes, so it is now offered as standard treatment to these patients (see chapter 10).

BREAST CANCER

Breast cancer accounts for approximately 14 percent of cancer incidence, and 9 percent of cancer mortality, in the United States. It is the most common cancer among women, and it is estimated that about 1 in every 10 women will develop breast cancer at some point in life. Breast cancer also occurs in men, but is more than a hundred-fold less frequent than in women.

Some rare forms of breast cancer are directly inherited, as discussed in chapter 6. In addition, the overall risk of developing breast cancer is increased two- or three-fold for women whose mothers or sisters have had the disease, presumably reflecting inherited disease susceptibility (see chapter 6). Furthermore, women who have had one breast cancer are at higher than average risk of developing a second. Other risk factors for breast cancer relate principally to the effects of hormones on the breast tissue. Breast cancer risk is increased about two-fold for women who have never had children, or who had their first child after age 35. In addition, early menarche (before age 12) or late menopause (after age 55) is associated with up to 1.5-fold increases in breast cancer risk. Oral contraceptive use is not associated with a significant overall increase in breast cancer incidence, although use of birth control pills for several years prior to first pregnancy may result in a modest increase in risk. Long-term postmenopausal estrogen replacement therapy may also be associated with a modest increase (less than 1.5-fold) in breast cancer risk, but this has not been definitively established. In addition, obesity may increase the risk of breast cancer up to 1.5-fold.

There are several different types of breast carcinomas. The majority (nearly 90%) arise in the ducts (Fig. 14.3) and are called ductal carcinomas. They are further distinguished according to cell type. The most common is called invasive ductal, NOS (for "not otherwise specified"). Other types of ductal carcinomas are medullary, tubular, and mucinous. About 5 percent of breast cancers arise in the lobules and are called lobular carcinomas. The remainder are classified as Paget's disease, which involves the nipple; and inflammatory carcinomas, which are associated with apparent inflammation of the breast.

Breast cancers frequently involve the *RB* and *p53* tumor suppressor genes, as well as c-*myc* and *erb*B-2 oncogenes. Expression of *erb*B-2, in particular, is more frequent in advanced-stage tumors and may be correlated with a less favorable prognosis (see chapter 7).

Early detection is of major importance in reducing breast cancer mortality, and screening for breast cancer by breast self-examination, examination by a physician, and mammography is recommended. It is

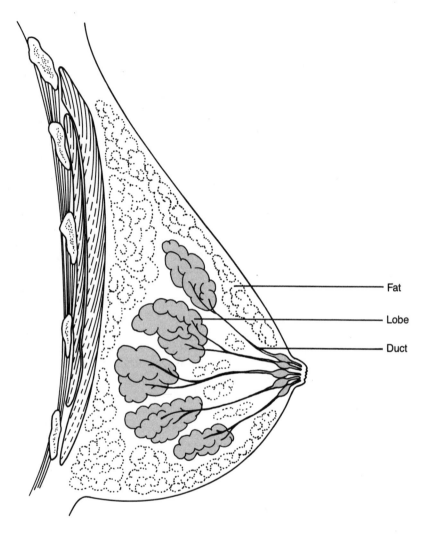

Figure 14.3

Cross-section of a breast.

estimated that annual screening by mammography for women over age 40 reduces breast cancer mortality by about 30 percent.

Breast cancers are treated by surgery and radiation, sometimes combined with chemotherapy and hormone therapy. For early-stage localized cancers, it is now often possible to remove only the tumor, rather than the entire breast. Radiation is then used to eliminate remaining cancer cells. Chemotherapy and hormone therapy may be used as adjuvants for treatment of localized disease, as well as for control of metastatic tumors. Hormone therapy with tamoxifen (an antiestrogen) is frequently effective in controlling the growth of tumors that express estrogen and progesterone receptors, so it is important to determine whether these receptors are present on tumor samples obtained at biopsy.

The benefits of early detection are apparent in terms of survival rates. The cure rate for carcinoma *in situ* is virtually 100 percent, and for localized invasive cancer, 90 percent. The survival rate drops to about 70 percent for disease that has spread to regional lymph nodes, however, and to less than 20 percent once metastasis to distant body sites has occurred.

PROSTATE CANCER

Cancer of the prostate (Fig. 14.4) accounts for approximately 10 percent of all cancer cases, and about 6 percent of total cancer mortality. It is the most common cancer in men; approximately 1 out of every 11 men will develop this disease.

The risk of prostate cancer, or adenocarcinoma, increases with age, and over 80 percent of prostate cancers occur in men past age 65. Possible causes and risk factors for the disease have not been established, although development of these cancers may involve stimulation of

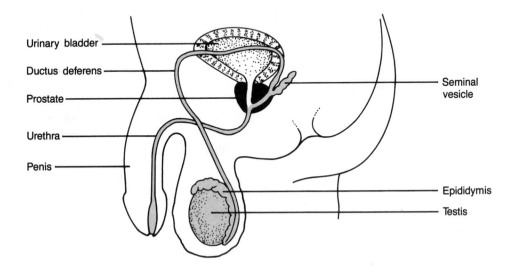

Figure 14.4

The male reproductive tract.

prostate cell proliferation by testosterone. Prostate carcinomas frequently involve mutations of the *RB* tumor suppressor gene.

Early detection plays a major role in reducing mortality from prostate cancer. The most effective screen for prostate cancer is a rectal exam, which should be performed annually for men over the age of 40. Ultrasonography and blood tests for prostate-specific antigen (see chapter 9) are being evaluated as additional early-detection methods. Symptoms, which may not occur in early stages of the disease, include problems in urination and persistent pain in the lower back, hips, or pelvis.

The five-year survival rate for prostate cancer is about 70 percent. More than half of prostate cancers are diagnosed while the disease is still localized, and the cure rate for these patients is over 80 percent. Except for very small tumors, surgical treatment usually involves removal of the entire prostate gland and surrounding tissue. Impotence, resulting from nerve damage, used to be a nearly universal side effect of this procedure, but improved surgical techniques now result in the recovery of potency in 50 to 80 percent of patients. For localized prostate cancer, radiation therapy is an alternative to surgery, and usually preserves potency. More advanced stages of prostate cancer are treated by hormone therapy. As discussed in chapter 10, the growth of prostate cancer cells is dependent on testosterone, and several kinds of hormone therapy may be employed to block hormonal stimulation of the cancer cells. These treatments include removal of the testes (orchiectomy) or administration of estrogen, analogs of gonadotropin-releasing hormone, or antiandrogens. Hormone therapy is not curative, but usually slows disease progression, relieves symptoms, and prolongs the lives of most patients.

URINARY CANCERS

Urinary cancers account for a total of approximately 7 percent of cancer incidence and 4 percent of mortality. About two-thirds of these cancers arise in the bladder, with most of the remainder being cancers of the kidney (Fig. 14.5).

Almost all bladder cancers originate from the transitional epithelium of the bladder, and are therefore called transitional cell carcinomas. Bladder cancer occurs primarily at age 60 and above, and is nearly three times more frequent in men than in women. Smoking results in about a two-fold increase in bladder cancer risk. Occupational exposure to dyes, rubber, and leather are additional risk factors. Contrary to early concerns, artificial sweeteners and coffee drinking do not appear to be associated with increased bladder cancer incidence. Mutations of the *RB* and *p53* tumor suppressor genes occur frequently in bladder carcinomas.

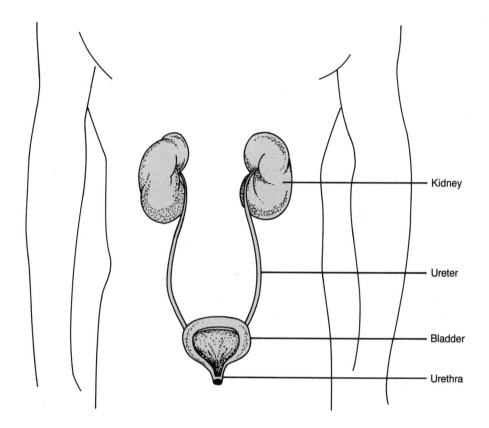

Kidney

Ureter

Bladder

Urethra

Figure 14.5

The urinary system.

The primary symptom of bladder cancer is blood in the urine. Diagnosis is usually by examination of the bladder by cystoscopy. The primary treatment is surgery, either alone or in combination with radiation or chemotherapy. The cure rate is nearly 90 percent for patients with localized disease. For patients with regional disease, survival is about 40 percent, and for patients with distant metastases, about 10 percent. It is noteworthy that favorable responses in over 50 percent of patients with advanced disease have recently been obtained by combination chemotherapy with the drugs methotrexate, vinblastine, doxorubicin, and cisplatin. The efficacy of this regimen, which may represent a significant treatment advance, is undergoing further evaluation.

Kidney cancer, like bladder cancer, is more frequent among men than women, and smoking is associated with about a two-fold increase in risk. Obesity is also a risk factor for women, possibly associated with excess estrogen production.

Early detection of kidney cancer is difficult, since early stages of the disease produce no clear signs or symptoms. The disease may be suggested by a variety of symptoms, including blood in the urine, pain in the side, abdomen, or back, weight loss, and weakness. Diagnosis is made by a variety of imaging techniques. The overall survival rate is about 40 percent, with surgery being the primary treatment. Prognosis is good for disease that remains localized to the kidney but poor for patients with disseminated disease.

UTERINE CANCERS

Cancers of the uterus (Fig. 14.6) account for approximately 4 percent of total cancer incidence and 2 percent of mortality. Cancers of this organ include two distinct types: cancers of the cervix and cancers of the endometrium.

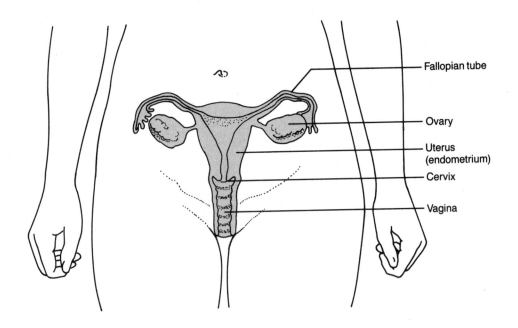

Fallopian tube

Ovary

Uterus
(endometrium)

Cervix

Vagina

Figure 14.6

The female reproductive tract.

Cervical cancer—usually squamous cell carcinoma—is responsible for about 30 percent of uterine cancer cases and about 60 percent of deaths. As discussed in chapter 5, most cases of cervical cancer are associated with human papillomaviruses, which are sexually transmitted. The major risk factors for cervical cancer are, therefore, associated with sexual practices such as intercourse with multiple partners. Cigarette smoking also appears to be associated with an increased disease incidence.

Early detection by the Pap smear has been extremely effective against cervical cancer. As discussed in chapter 9, very early stages of disease can be reliably detected by this method. Presently, about 50,000 cases of cervical carcinoma *in situ* are detected annually by the Pap test. These cases are not included in the incidence and mortality figures given above, which are based on the 13,500 cases of cervical carcinoma per year that remain undetected until more advanced stages. Thus, screening by the Pap smear currently detects over 75 percent of cervical carcinomas before they become invasive, and the use of regular screening could be expected to prevent development of most of the remaining invasive cases of this disease.

Cervical cancer is treated by surgery or radiation. The cure rate for carcinoma *in situ* is virtually 100 percent following minor procedures, and localized carcinoma remains curable in nearly 90 percent of cases. Survival rates for disease that has spread regionally, however, drop to about 50 percent, and fall to below 20 percent for metastatic cancers. The key to effective reduction in mortality from this disease, therefore, remains early detection.

Endometrial cancer, usually adenocarcinoma, accounts for about 70 percent of uterine cancers excluding cervical carcinomas *in situ*. The risk factors for endometrial cancer involve excess stimulation of endometrial cell proliferation by estrogen in the absence of progesterone. Obesity increases endometrial cancer risk several-fold, most likely as a result of estrogen production by fat cells. Other risk factors are failure to ovulate and a history of infertility, which may also be associated with an estrogen imbalance. In addition, the risk of endometrial cancer is increased by long-term (greater than one year) postmenopausal estrogen replacement therapy with high doses of estrogen alone. However, this risk is minimized by the use of lower doses of estrogen in combination with progesterone, which counteracts the stimulatory effect of estrogen on endometrial cell proliferation. The birth control pills currently available contain progesterone as well as estrogen, and appear to result in a reduced, rather than increased, risk of endometrial cancer.

Unfortunately, the Pap smear is only partially effective in diagnosis of endometrial cancer, and this disease is not usually detected until symptoms are evident. The disease is most common in women between the ages of 55 and 70, and the American Cancer Society recommends that women at increased risk (e.g., with a history of infertility or obesity) have an endometrial biopsy at menopause. Patients receiving estrogen replacement therapy should have endometrial biopsies repeated periodically. The most common symptom of the disease after menopause is vaginal bleeding.

Diagnosis of endometrial cancer is by biopsy or dilation and curettage (D and C). Surgery and radiotherapy are effective in treatment of localized disease, and survival rates for these patients are over 90 percent. Regional spread of disease outside of the uterus is still treatable by radiation, with survival rates in excess of 65 percent. Advanced, metastatic endometrial cancer is generally treated by administration of progesterone, which results in prolonged survival, although not cures, in about one-third of patients. The overall survival rate for endometrial cancer is about 85 percent.

ORAL CANCERS

Oral cancers, including cancers of the lip, tongue, mouth, and pharynx (Figs. 14.1 and 14.2), account for approximately 3 percent of cancer incidence and 1.6 percent of mortality. Cancers at these sites are usually squamous cell carcinomas. The major risk factors for oral cancers are tobacco use and excess consumption of alcoholic beverages, particularly in combination. As a consequence of such carcinogen exposure, patients with one such cancer are at high risk of developing a second, independent tumor. Excessive exposure to sunlight is also an important risk factor for lip cancer.

The genetic alterations involved in oral cancers have not been well characterized. However, given the relationship of these tumors to tobacco carcinogens, they might be expected to involve some of the same types of carcinogen-related events found in lung cancers, such as mutations of the *p53* tumor suppressor gene.

Early detection is important in the prognosis of oral cancers, and is best accomplished by regular examination of the mouth and throat by dentists and physicians. Leukoplakia, which may be observed during such an examination, is a white patch (*leuko* = white, and *plakia* = patch) on a mucous membrane of the mouth. Sometimes, but not always, leukoplakia represents either a preneoplastic cell proliferation or a more advanced stage of carcinoma development. Following biopsy, approximately 10 percent of patients with leukoplakia are diagnosed with preneoplastic dysplasias or carcinoma *in situ*, and approximately 5 percent with invasive carcinoma.

Treatment of oral cancers is primarily by surgery or radiotherapy. The overall survival rate for these cancers is about 50 percent, depending on the site and stage of disease. The survival rate for lip cancer, for example, is about 90 percent, while that for cancer of the pharynx is approximately 30 percent.

PANCREATIC CANCER

Cancer of the pancreas, an adenocarcinoma, accounts for approximately 3 percent of cancer incidence and 5 percent of mortality. Most cases occur after age 65. Cigarette smoking, which increases pancreatic cancer incidence about two-fold, is the only known risk factor. Nearly 90 percent of these cancers involve *ras* oncogenes.

There is currently no early detection method for pancreatic cancer, and the disease produces no symptoms until it reaches advanced stages. Treatment is ineffective; the five-year survival rate is only 3 percent.

MELANOMA AND OTHER SKIN CANCERS

Melanoma is a cancer arising from pigment-producing cells in the skin. It accounts for approximately 2.6 percent of cancer incidence and 1.2 percent of mortality. The incidence of melanoma throughout the world has been steadily increasing for the last forty years.

The major risk factor for melanoma is ultraviolet radiation from sunlight. It is about ten times more frequent among white people than among black people, presumably because the greater pigmentation of dark skin protects against radiation. In rare cases, familial susceptibility to melanoma may be inherited, for example, in individuals with dysplastic nevus syndrome or xeroderma pigmentosum (see chapter 6).

Early detection is critical to the outcome of melanoma, and is best accomplished by self-examination of the skin. Melanomas may develop within a mole, or as a new molelike growth. They are characterized by increasing size and changes in color (Fig. 14.7). The American Cancer Society emphasizes four warning signs of melanoma: (1) assymetry, meaning the shape of one half of a mole is different from the other, (2) border irregularities, such as uneven, ragged, or notched edges, (3) different colors within a mole, and (4) size greater than 6 mm (about 1/4″) in diameter.

Treatment of melanoma is primarily surgical removal, possibly including excision of regional lymph nodes. Survival rates are about 90 percent for localized melanoma, but metastatic disease is not responsive to

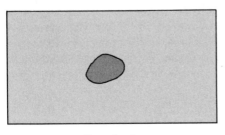

Normal mole

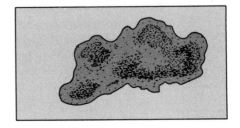

Melanoma

Figure 14.7

Comparison of a normal mole and a melanoma. Melanomas are characterized by increasing size and irregularities in shape, border, and coloration.

therapy. Since melanomas can metastasize quickly, early detection is the major determinant of prognosis.

The nonmelanoma skin cancers—basal cell and squamous cell carcinomas—are extremely common but seldom lethal. For this reason, these cancers are generally not included in calculations of cancer incidence, including those in this chapter. Nonmelanoma skin cancers, like melanoma, are caused by solar ultraviolet radiation. In contrast to melanoma, however, basal cell and squamous cell carcinomas metastasize very slowly. They are consequently readily cured by surgery or radiation. There are estimated to be more than 600,000 cases of nonmelanoma skin cancers diagnosed each year, but they result in only about 2,500 deaths—a cure rate of approximately 99.5 percent.

STOMACH CANCER

Stomach cancer (adenocarcinoma) accounts for approximately 2 percent of United States cancer incidence and 2.7 percent of mortality, although it is much more common in other parts of the world. For example, stomach cancer in Japan is about five times more common than in the United States. It is also noteworthy that, as discussed in chapter 1, stomach cancer in the United States has declined more than five-fold since 1930.

Excessive consumption of cured, smoked, and pickled foods, which contain large amounts of salt, nitrates, and nitrites, is thought to be a major risk factor for stomach cancer. As discussed in chapters 4 and 8, nitrates and nitrites are converted to potent carcinogens, nitrosamines. Vitamin C blocks the formation of nitrosamines, and may be responsible for the protective effect of fresh fruits and vegetables against stomach cancer. The decline in stomach cancer in this country is thought to be the result of refrigeration for food preservation, correlated with a decreased use of cured and smoked foods, as well as increased consumption of fresh fruits and vegetables.

Early detection of stomach cancer is difficult, since symptoms frequently do not develop until the disease is relatively advanced. Symptoms include indigestion, abdominal discomfort, loss of appetite, and weight loss. Diagnosis involves x-rays and gastroscopy. Surgery is the primary treatment, which may be combined with radiation or chemotherapy. Surgery is potentially curative only for localized disease, however, and overall survival rates are only 15 percent.

OVARIAN CANCER

Cancer of the ovary (see Fig. 14.6) accounts for approximately 2 percent of cancer incidence and 2.4 percent of mortality. About 90 percent of ovarian cancers are adenocarcinomas arising from the epithelial cells covering the ovary. There are four major types of these tumors: (1) serous, (2) mucinous, (3) endometrioid, and (4) clear-cell. Relatively infrequently ovarian tumors arise from germ cells (dysgerminomas, yolk-sac carcinomas, teratomas, and choriocarcinomas) or from other ovarian cell types, such as granulosa, theca, and Sertoli-Leydig cells.

The risk of ovarian cancer appears to be affected primarily by reproductive history, indicating that hormonal factors are important in its development. Women who have not had children have about a two-fold increased risk of developing ovarian cancer, but the risk decreases to below average for women who have had several pregnancies. Birth control pills, which, like pregnancy, prevent ovulation, also appear to decrease ovarian cancer risk. In addition, women who have breast or endometrial cancers are about twice as likely to develop ovarian cancer. Ovarian cancers frequently involve mutations of the *p53* tumor suppressor gene. As discussed in chapter 7, the erbB-2 oncogene also plays an important role in progression to more aggressive tumor growth.

Ovarian cancer is usually asymptomatic until relatively advanced stages, and it is not detected by the Pap test. Early detection is best accomplished through periodic pelvic examinations, but the majority of ovarian carcinomas have already reached an advanced stage by the time of diagnosis. Ultrasonography and tests for an ovarian tumor marker, called CA-125, in the blood are being evaluated as possible screening methods. Common symptoms are abdominal swelling and bloating. Treatment includes surgery, radiation, and chemotherapy. The survival rate for localized disease is over 80 percent, but drops to 45 percent for cancers that have spread beyond the ovary, and to less than 20 percent once metastasis to distant sites has occurred. Overall, the five-year survival rate for ovarian cancer is 38 percent.

BRAIN TUMORS

Brain tumors account for approximately 1.5 percent of adult cancer incidence and 2.2 percent of mortality. As indicated for childhood brain tumors in chapter 13, causes and risk factors are unknown. There are many different types of brain cancers, the most prevalent in adults being astrocytomas, ependymomas, and meningiomas. Astrocytomas and ependymomas are malignant, whereas meningiomas are benign. Astrocytomas, which include glioblastomas, account for about 50 percent of adult brain tumors. These tumors frequently involve mutations of the *p53* tumor suppressor gene.

Headaches are the most common symptom of adult brain tumors, which are then diagnosed by a variety of imaging techniques, such as computed tomography (CT scan) and magnetic resonance imaging (MRI), as well as electroencephalography (EEG). The standard treatment is surgery, often combined with radiation and chemotherapy. The overall survival rate is under 30 percent, but this varies considerably according to tumor type and location. Even benign brain tumors, such as meningiomas, are not always curable, since their location may preclude complete surgical removal.

LIVER CANCER

Cancers of the liver and gall bladder (see Fig. 14.2) constitute about 1.4 percent of United States cancer incidence and 2.3 percent of mortality. The primary cause of liver cancer is infection with hepatitis B virus, and the disease is much more common in other parts of the world, where infection with this virus is prevalent (see chapter 5). Aflatoxin is also a potent liver carcinogen, which is produced by a fungus that frequently contaminates poorly stored peanuts and other foods. The level of aflatoxin allowed in peanut butter is carefully controlled in the United States, but aflatoxin contamination of foodstuffs is associated with high rates of liver cancer in other countries. Cirrhosis, which can be caused by excess alcohol consumption, is also correlated with an increased risk of liver cancer. Mutations of the *p53* tumor suppressor gene, possibly resulting from the action of aflatoxin (see chapter 7), are frequently found in liver cancers.

Symptoms of liver cancer are pain, weight loss, loss of appetite, and fatigue. The disease may be treated by surgery, radiation, and chemotherapy. Prognosis is poor, however, and the five-year survival rate is only 4 percent.

LARYNGEAL CANCER

Cancer of the larynx (see Fig. 14.1) accounts for 1.2 percent of cancer incidence and 0.7 percent of mortality. Laryngeal cancers are squamous cell carcinomas, which, like lung cancer, are primarily caused by cigarette smoking. As in the case of oral cancers, excess alcohol consumption, particularly in combination with smoking, may also increase laryngeal cancer risk.

Hoarseness is an early symptom of laryngeal cancer, and persistent hoarseness should be evaluated by a physician. Additional symptoms include pain or sore throats. Diagnosis is by examination with a laryngoscope. The primary treatment for laryngeal cancer is surgery or radiotherapy. Radiation is the preferred treatment for localized laryngeal cancers, since loss of speech is prevented thereby. The overall survival rate for patients with laryngeal cancer is 68 percent.

THYROID CANCER

Cancers of the thyroid gland account for about 1 percent of cancer incidence and 0.2 percent of mortality. There are four major histological types: (1) papillary, (2) follicular, (3) medullary, and (4) anaplastic. Papillary carcinomas are the most common, accounting for over 50 percent of all thyroid cancers. Some medullary carcinomas are inherited as part of multiple endocrine neoplasia types 2A and 2B (see chapter 6). The major environmental risk factor for thyroid cancer is radiation. More specifically, childhood exposure to radiation of the head and neck as therapy for such conditions as enlarged thymus or tonsils is associated with a subsequent increased incidence of thyroid carcinomas. Radiation was a common treatment for these conditions prior to the 1950s, but it is no longer used. Several oncogenes are regularly involved in papillary thyroid carcinomas, including the *ras* genes.

Thyroid carcinomas are usually detected as a lump during physical examination. The primary treatment is surgery, frequently in combination with administration of radioactive iodine, a source of radiation that localizes in the thyroid gland and may serve to eliminate residual cancer cells. The prognosis for most patients with thyroid cancer is excellent, and survival rates are greater than 90 percent. An exception is anaplastic carcinoma, which represents approximately 20 percent of all thyroid carcinomas. Five-year survival rates for patients with this disease are less than 10 percent.

ESOPHAGEAL CANCER

Cancer of the esophagus (see Fig. 14.2) accounts for about 1 percent of cancer incidence and nearly 2 percent of mortality. Cancers of this site are usually squamous cell carcinomas. The major risk factors for esophageal cancer are the same as for oral cancers: tobacco and excess alcohol consumption. The *p53* tumor suppressor gene is frequently mutated in esophageal carcinomas.

The most common symptom of esophageal cancer is difficulty in swallowing, but the disease has frequently progressed to an advanced state before symptoms are evident. Surgery and radiotherapy are the principal treatments, but the prognosis for patients with esophageal cancer is poor, corresponding to a five-year survival rate of 8 percent.

TESTICULAR CANCER

Cancer of the testes (see Fig. 14.4) accounts for about 0.6 percent of total cancer incidence and less than 0.1 percent of mortality. The causes of testicular cancer are unknown, but men between the ages of 20 and 35 are at the greatest risk. The disease is usually detected as a lump on the testis, either during self-examination or by a physician.

There are several different types of testicular cancer, nearly all of which arise from germ cells within the testis. Seminomas, which account for approximately 40 percent of all testicular cancers, are composed of morphologically undifferentiated cells. The nonseminomatous testicular cancers, which include choriocarcinomas, embryonal carcinomas, teratomas, and yolk-sac carcinomas, contain more specialized cell types.

Seminomas are usually detected at an early stage, when they are still localized. In addition, these tumors are particularly sensitive to radiation. Consequently, treatment of seminomas with a combination of surgery + radiotherapy is curative for more than 90 percent of patients.

The nonseminomatous testicular cancers, on the other hand, are usually not detected until they have progressed to a more advanced stage of disease and, in most cases, these tumors have already metastasized by the time of diagnosis. Nonetheless, recent advances in chemotherapy have made these highly treatable forms of cancer. In particular, these tumors are unusually sensitive to the drug cisplatin. Treatment of nonseminomatous testicular cancers is therefore usually surgery + combination chemotherapy. A common drug combination is cisplatin, bleomycin, and vinblastine. Survival rates for nonseminomatous testicular cancers are in excess of 75 percent, and survival rates for all testicular cancers combined are over 90 percent.

SUMMARY

The solid tumors discussed in this chapter comprise about 85 percent of United States cancer incidence and 81 percent of mortality. Together with the leukemias and lymphomas (8% of incidence and 9% of mortality), these diseases account for over 90 percent of the cancer burden in this country, the remainder being sarcomas (approximately 1% of both incidence and mortality) and comparatively infrequent carcinomas of other sites. The major risk factors for these cancers include tobacco, alcohol, diet, radiation, estrogen imbalances, and viruses. A variety of oncogenes and tumor suppressor genes are involved in these tumors, often with multiple genes contributing in a cumulative fashion to the development of malignancy.

In most cases, the survival rates for adult patients with solid tumors are determined by the stage at which cancer is diagnosed. In general, localized cancers can be successfully treated, but therapy is much less effective once the cancer has spread from its site of origin. Hence, early diagnosis is often the major determinant of disease outcome.

PART V

Prospects for the Future

Chapter 15

The War on Cancer—
Progress and Promises

Cancer has been with us throughout human history and has long been a focus of medical practice. Indeed, the term *carcinoma* was coined by Hippocrates in the fourth century B.C., and efforts to deal with the cancer problem have been ongoing since that time. Some of the notable events in the battle against cancer during the last two centuries include the first association between the use of tobacco (snuff) and cancer in 1761, identification of the first occupational carcinogen (chimney soot) in 1775, the first surgical cure of an abdominal tumor in 1809 (the patient survived thirty years after removal of a twenty-two-pound ovarian carcinoma), the discovery of tumor viruses in 1908, identification of the first chemical carcinogen (coal tar) in 1915, the development of the Pap test in 1928, the first successful chemotherapy of childhood leukemia in 1947, and the Report of the Surgeon General on Smoking and Health in 1964.

It was against this historical background that President Richard M. Nixon signed the National Cancer Act in 1971, declaring the start of the so-called War on Cancer. The prevention and treatment of cancer were obviously already areas of intense research, but the notion of a "war on cancer" focused public attention on the cancer problem as a top national priority. Twenty years later, it seems reasonable to ask how we are doing.

The War on Cancer has been fought on two fronts, which, to date, have remained largely distinct efforts. Practical efforts have focused on cancer prevention and treatment, while major basic research efforts have been directed at understanding cancer at the cellular and molecular levels. It is all too clear that cancer has not been conquered, but significant advances in the prevention and treatment of cancer have been made. Moreover, progress in understanding the fundamental mechanisms responsible for the development of cancer has been dramatic. Major improvements in our ability to deal with cancer may eventually result from applying our increasing understanding of cancer's molecular basis to the development of new strategies for cancer prevention and treatment.

PROGRESS IN CANCER PREVENTION AND TREATMENT

Some critics of the War on Cancer have asserted that there has been little progress in dealing with cancer, since there has been no significant decrease in overall cancer deaths. Although the likelihood of dying from cancer is the ultimate bottom line, this seems to be too dismissive a position—it ignores the progress that has been made. Although far from representing the successful conquest of cancer, such progress is significant and needs to be understood in the context of the overall cancer problem.

First, it is important to emphasize that we already have knowledge at hand that could prevent a significant fraction of cancer deaths, but these preventive measures are not being effectively applied. Significant progress has been made both in the identification of the causes of certain cancers and in the detection of some cancers at early, more treatable, stages of the disease process. The translation of these findings into significant reductions in cancer mortality, however, involves changes in lifestyles, which are difficult to implement. In addition, it is important to realize that, because of the characteristically long lag time between carcinogen exposure and tumor development, the effects of preventive measures on overall cancer mortality often are not evident for several decades after their implementation.

Most notably, about one-third of cancer deaths in the United States could be eliminated by avoidance of tobacco. This realization has led to a reduction in the prevalence of smoking, but hardly to its elimination. About 40 percent of American adults smoked in 1965, and about 30 percent still smoke today, including many teenagers. Even twenty years after its identification as a major cause of cancer, the use of tobacco remains a problem. Thus, while the elimination of tobacco use has the potential of making a major impact against cancer, this has not yet been realized. Apparently, the prospect of cancer prevention is not a strong enough motivation for many members of our society to avoid tobacco use.

Given the limited impact of knowledge that tobacco is a major carcinogen, it is difficult to be optimistic about the possibility of cancer prevention based on voluntary changes in lifestyle. Thus, although alcohol, obesity, high-fat diets, and sexually-transmitted viruses are clearly risk factors for some cancers, it seems unlikely that cancer prevention is a sufficient motivation for many people to alter their behavior and reduce their risk accordingly. Recent studies of dietary factors, for example, indicate that colon cancer incidence might be halved by reducing dietary fat intake from 40 percent to 30 percent of total calories. Such a change in eating habits throughout the United States could be expected to reduce total cancer mortality by about 5 percent, but the widespread adoption of a major dietary modification to achieve this relatively modest reduction in cancer risk must be considered unlikely. Similar motivational problems appear to apply to the widespread acceptance of early screening tests, which could reduce overall cancer mortality by about another 10 percent. It appears that the majority of exposures to carcinogens are determined by personal lifestyle choices rather than factors such as industrial pollution. Consequently, voluntary modifications of behavior will be needed to achieve any significant reduction in cancer mortality based on preventive measures.

Nonetheless, this should not obscure the fact that significant progress has been made in identifying the causes of several cancers, and in detecting some cancers at early, readily treatable stages. If current recommendations for cancer prevention and early detection were put into general practice, they would result in about a two-fold reduction in total cancer mortality. This would clearly represent substantial progress, suggesting that the most effective step that can currently be taken against cancer is to increase public awareness and motivation in order to take advantage of what we already know in the area of cancer prevention.

The discovery of viruses as the causes of some cancers affords an alternative approach to prevention, namely the development of antiviral vaccines. Indeed, a safe and apparently effective vaccine against hepatitis B virus is already in use and can be reasonably expected to have a significant impact on the incidence of liver cancer. Although rare in the United States, liver cancer is extremely common in parts of Asia and Africa, probably accounting for about 10 percent of total worldwide cancer incidence. Its potential prevention by a vaccination program thus represents a major step in the international cancer effort.

Progress has also been made in the treatment of some cancers, although not for those that are most common in our society. For the majority of cancers, the success of treatment is primarily determined by early diagnosis. Localized cancers can be frequently cured by surgery and radiation, but chemotherapy of metastatic disease usually fails. However, drug combinations have now been developed that are capable of curing most patients suffering from acute lymphocytic leukemia, Hodgkin's disease, some non-Hodgkin's lymphomas, and testicular cancer. But together, these diseases account for less than 5 percent of the total cancer burden, so their successful treatment has not made a significant impact on overall cancer statistics. On the other hand, these successes are real, and they suggest that similar progress against other cancers is within the realm of possibility. Indeed, the activity of fluorouracil + levamisole against colon cancer (see chapter 10) represents a recent example of at least modest progress in the treatment of one of the most common cancers of adults.

Significant progress in some types of immunotherapy has also been made, although this has not yet been translated into general practice. Specific populations of antitumor lymphocytes have been identified, and they have been shown to have significant therapeutic effects in early-stage clinical trials against melanomas and kidney cancers. Moreover, experiments are currently underway to use genetic engineering to make these lymphocytes even more potent killers of cancer cells. Success along these avenues could lead to significant advances in cancer treatments in the future.

In summary, real progress against cancer has been made, but practical advances have been slow and efforts to date have not led to any significant decrease in cancer deaths. Public education, to effectively implement currently understood preventive measures (particularly avoidance of tobacco), would have the greatest immediate impact on cancer mortality. Advances in chemotherapy have led to successes against a few malignancies, but not against the majority of common cancers.

PROGRESS IN UNDERSTANDING CANCER

In contrast to the relatively slow progress in cancer prevention and treatment, the last twenty years have seen dramatic advances in our understanding of cancer at the cellular and molecular levels. The discoveries of oncogenes and tumor suppressor genes have provided a conceptual framework for understanding the mechanisms that control normal cell growth and differentiation, and the ways in which breakdowns of these normal cellular controls lead to the development of cancer.

A large number of oncogenes and tumor suppressor genes have now been identified, and it is clear that mutations in these genes are fundamental to the development of human cancers. Many of these genes have been characterized with respect to their roles in regulating normal cell growth, and we have begun to understand how their malfunction can lead to the uncontrolled proliferation of cancer cells. Moreover, pictures of the ways in which multiple oncogenes and tumor suppressor genes are involved in the development of different types of human cancers are beginning to emerge.

Our understanding of the molecular and cellular basis of cancer has thus advanced tremendously, and progress in this area continues at a rapid pace. In addition to illuminating the mechanisms involved in abnormal tumor-cell growth, studies at this level have also resulted in substantial gains in our understanding of the basic mechanisms that regulate normal cell growth and differentiation. The current challenge, however, is to apply these newfound insights to the practical arenas of cancer prevention and treatment.

THE FUTURE'S PROMISE: WILL OUR UNDERSTANDING OF CANCER YIELD PRACTICAL BENEFITS?

There is little question that our increasing understanding of cancer will ultimately have an impact on diagnosis and treatment, but it is uncertain how profound this impact will be. It is already evident that oncogenes and tumor suppressor genes will be useful markers for the diagnosis of some cancers and thereby contribute to improvements in both early detection and therapy. Several examples are readily apparent and are already being put into clinical practice. Analysis of tumor suppressor genes will allow identification of individuals at high risk for inherited cancers. Detection of the *abl* oncogene in chronic myelogenous leukemia provides a sensitive assay for leukemic cells, which is useful in monitoring the response of patients to therapy. Expression of the N-*myc* oncogene in neuroblastomas, and of the *erb*B-2 oncogene in breast and ovarian carcinomas, is predictive of rapid disease progression, and may contribute to decisions between treatment options for patients with these diseases. Ongoing research in this area will undoubtedly identify diagnostic roles for additional genes in other cancers. However, although this information will be useful and may well lead to improvements in diagnosis and subsequent treatment, it is not likely to have a major impact on the overall cancer problem. In the end, we will still be limited by the problems inherent in current treatment methods.

As discussed in chapter 10, the limitation of current chemotherapeutic drugs is that they are not specific for cancer cells. Instead, the present chemotherapeutic agents interfere nonspecifically with cell division, and are, therefore, toxic to rapidly proliferating normal cells as well as to cancer cells. This toxicity to normal cells limits the effectiveness of chemotherapy—a problem that could be overcome if drugs specific for cancer cells could be found. Can the discoveries of oncogenes and tumor suppressor genes be exploited to provide such specific targets against which a new generation of anticancer drugs might act? Is it possible, for example, to design drugs that specifically interfere with the function of oncogene proteins, or that augment the activity of tumor suppressor gene products?

Unfortunately from the standpoint of cancer chemotherapy, oncogenes and tumor suppressor genes are important in normal cells as well as in cancer cells. Since the products of these genes are critical regulators of normal cell proliferation, they do not provide chemotherapeutic targets that are unique to cancer cells. Consequently, the possible exploitation of oncogenes and tumor suppressor genes in the treatment of cancer is not a straightforward proposition, but there are also reasons to hope that it will not ultimately be an impossible one.

One example that illustrates the possibility of such an oncogene-directed therapy, discussed in chapters 10 and 12, is the treatment of acute promyelocytic leukemia with retinoic acid. In this disease, the retinoic-acid receptor is mutated so that it acts as an oncogene, most likely by interfering with the ability of the normal receptor to induce cell differentiation. Strikingly, the disease can be treated by administration of retinoic acid, which appears to compensate for the aberrant receptor and induce differentiation of the leukemic cells. Although the mechanisms involved are not yet fully elucidated, this seems to be a clear case of an effective cancer treatment directed against a specific oncogene.

Our understanding of the relationships between hormones, growth factors, tumor suppressor genes, and oncogenes is growing rapidly, and may well suggest similar manipulations of hormones and growth factors for the treatment of other tumors. Thus, the development of drugs that affect specific growth-control pathways, and their rational use based on the oncogenes and tumor suppressor genes involved in particular types of cancer, seem to represent a plausible area of future developments in cancer therapy. A great deal of further work will clearly be required, but this approach appears to at least offer the promise of developing drugs that are specifically targeted towards cancer cells. If such drugs were nontoxic, their use in chemoprevention could also be considered. Indeed, as discussed in chapter 8, chemoprevention trials of retinoic acid derivatives and tamoxifen are already in progress.

SUMMARY

Although we are far from the ultimate conquest of cancer, major advances have been made. The greatest immediate impact on cancer mortality could be attained by public adoption of the lifestyle changes required to eliminate major carcinogens, most notably tobacco, and to maximize the benefits of early detection. Chemotherapy has proven successful against a few relatively rare cancers, but not so far against the more common malignancies. On the other hand, striking progress has been made in understanding cancer at the molecular and cellular levels. The challenge of the future, which may well determine the ultimate success of the War on Cancer, is to apply this understanding to the practical matters of cancer prevention and treatment.

Appendix

Information and Resources for Cancer Patients

AMERICAN CANCER SOCIETY, INC.
1599 Clifton Road, N.E.
Atlanta, Georgia 30329
800–ACS–2345

The American Cancer Society is a national voluntary organization that supports cancer research and offers a variety of services for cancer patients, including information, counseling, and rehabilitation programs. Educational programs include distribution of a number of pamphlets and booklets on cancer. Local American Cancer Society units provide counseling, home care items, and transportation for cancer patients.

Additional national rehabilitation and education programs are:

CanSurmount: A short-term visitor program for cancer patients and their families. One-on-one visits offer support by an individual who has experienced the same type of cancer as the patient.

I Can Cope: A series of lectures and group discussions covering the concerns of cancer patients and their families.

Laryngectomy Rehabilitation: The International Association of Laryngectomees is a group of more than 250 clubs that provide support for laryngectomy patients.

Look Good—Feel Better: A program designed to help patients develop cosmetic skills to improve their appearance and deal with side-effects of cancer treatment.

Ostomy Rehabilitation: A support program, in cooperation with the United Ostomy Association, to help patients with urinary or intestinal

203

cancers cope with ostomies. One-on-one counseling is provided by volunteers who have undergone the same type of surgery.

Reach to Recovery: A support program for women who have had mastectomies.

CHARTERED DIVISIONS OF THE AMERICAN CANCER SOCIETY

Alabama Division, Inc.
504 Brookwood Boulevard
Homewood, Alabama 35209
205-879-2242

Alaska Division, Inc.
406 West Fireweed Lane, Suite 204
Anchorage, Alaska 99503
907-277-8696

Arizona Division, Inc.
2929 East Thomas Road
Phoenix, Arizona 85016
602-224-0524

Arkansas Division, Inc.
901 North University
Little Rock, Arkansas 72207
501-664-3480

California Division, Inc.
1710 Webster Street
P.O. Box 2061
Oakland, California 94612
415-893-7900

Colorado Division, Inc.
2255 South Oneida
P.O. Box 24669
Denver, Colorado 80224
303-758-2030

Connecticut Division, Inc.
Barnes Park South
14 Village Lane
Wallingford, Connecticut 06492
203-265-7161

Delaware Division, Inc.
92 Read's Way
New Castle, Delaware 19720
302-324-4227

District of Columbia Division, Inc.
1825 Connecticut Avenue N.W.,
   Suite 315
Washington, D.C. 20009
202-483-2600

Florida Division, Inc.
1001 South MacDill Avenue
Tampa, Florida 33629
813-253-0541

Georgia Division, Inc.
46 Fifth Street N.E.
Atlanta, Georgia 30308
404-892-0026

Hawaii/Pacific Division, Inc.
Community Services Center Bldg.
200 North Vineyard Boulevard
Honolulu, Hawaii 96817
808-531-1662

Idaho Division, Inc.
2676 Vista Avenue
P.O. Box 5386
Boise, Idaho 83705
208-343-4609

Illinois Division, Inc.
77 East Monroe
Chicago, Illinois 60603
312-641-6150

Indiana Division, Inc.
8730 Commerce Park Place
Indianapolis, Indiana 46268
317–872–4432

Iowa Division, Inc.
8364 Hickman Road, Suite D
Des Moines, Iowa 50325
515–253–0147

Kansas Division, Inc.
1315 S.W. Arrowhead Road
Topeka, Kansas 66604
913–273–4114

Kentucky Division, Inc.
701 West Muhammad Ali Blvd.
P.O. Box 1807
Louisville, Kentucky 40201–1807
502–584–6782

Louisiana Division, Inc.
Fidelity Homestead Bldg.
837 Gravier Street, Suite 700
New Orleans, Louisiana 70112–1509
504–523–4188

Maine Division, Inc.
52 Federal Street
Brunswick, Maine 04011
207–729–3339

Maryland Division, Inc.
8219 Town Center Drive
White Marsh, Maryland 21162–0082
301–931–6868

Massachusetts Division, Inc.
247 Commonwealth Avenue
Boston, Massachusetts 02116
617–267–2650

Michigan Division, Inc.
1205 East Saginaw Street
Lansing, Michigan 48906
517–371–2920

Minnesota Division, Inc.
3316 West 66th Street
Minneapolis, Minnesota 55435
612–925–2772

Mississippi Division, Inc.
Lakeover Office Park
1380 Livingston Lane
Jackson, Mississippi 39213
601–362–8874

Missouri Division, Inc.
3322 American Avenue
Jefferson City, Missouri 65102
314–893–4800

Montana Division, Inc.
313 N. 32nd Street, Suite 1
Billings, Montana 59101
406–252–7111

Nebraska Division, Inc.
8502 West Center Road
Omaha, Nebraska 68124–5255
402–393–5800

Nevada Division, Inc.
1325 East Harmon
Las Vegas, Nevada 89119
702–798–6857

New Hampshire Division, Inc.
360 Route 101, Unit 501
Bedford, New Hampshire 03102–6800
603–472–8899

New Jersey Division, Inc.
2600 Route 1, CN 2201
North Brunswick, New Jersey 08902
201–297–8000

New Mexico Division, Inc.
5800 Lomas Blvd. N.E.
Albuquerque, New Mexico 87110
505–260–2105

New York Division, Inc.
6725 Lyons Street
P.O. Box 7
East Syracuse, New York 13057
315–437–7025

Long Island Division, Inc.
145 Pidgeon Hill Road
Huntington Station, New York
11746
516–385–9100

New York City Division, Inc.
19 West 56th Street
New York, New York 10019
212–586–8700

Queens Division, Inc.
112–25 Queens Boulevard
Forest Hills, New York 11375
718–263–2224

Westchester Division, Inc.
30 Glenn St.
White Plains, New York 10603
914–949–4800

North Carolina Division, Inc.
11 South Boylan Avenue, Suite 221
Raleigh, North Carolina 27603
919–834–8463

North Dakota Division, Inc.
123 Roberts Street
P.O. Box 426
Fargo, North Dakota 58107
701–232–1385

Ohio Division, Inc.
5555 Frantz Road
Dublin, Ohio 43017
614-889-9565

Oklahoma Division, Inc.
3000 United Founders Blvd.,
Suite 136
Oklahoma City, Oklahoma 73112
405–843–9888

Oregon Division, Inc.
0330 S.W. Curry
Portland, Oregon 97201
503–295–6422

Pennsylvania Division, Inc.
Route 422 & Sipe Avenue
P.O. Box 897
Hershey, Pennsylvania 17033–0897
717–533–6144

Philadelphia Division, Inc.
1422 Chestnut Street
Philadelphia, Pennsylvania 19102
215–665–2900

Puerto Rico Division, Inc.
Calle Alverio #577
Esquina Sargento Medina
Hato Rey, Puerto Rico 00918
809–764–2295

Rhode Island Division, Inc.
400 Main Street
Pawtucket, Rhode Island 02860
401–722–8480

South Carolina Division, Inc.
128 Stonemark Lane
Columbia, South Carolina 29210
803–750–1693

South Dakota Division, Inc.
4101 Carnegie Place
Sioux Falls, South Dakota 57106–2322
605–361–8277

Tennessee Division, Inc.
1315 Eighth Avenue South
Nashville, Tennessee 37203
615–255–1227

Texas Division, Inc.
2433 Ridgepoint Drive
Austin, Texas 78754
512–928–2262

Utah Division, Inc.
610 East South Temple
Salt Lake City, Utah 84102
801–322–0431

Vermont Division, Inc.
13 Loomis Street, Drawer C
P.O. Box 1452
Montpelier, Vermont 05601–1452
802–223–2348

Virginia Division, Inc.
4240 Park Place Court
Glen Allen, Virginia 23060
804–270–0142

Washington Division, Inc.
2120 First Avenue North
Seattle, Washington 98109–1140
206–283–1152

West Virginia Division, Inc.
2428 Kanawha Boulevard East
Charleston, West Virginia 25311
304–344–3611

Wisconsin Division, Inc.
615 North Sherman Avenue
Madison, Wisconsin 53704
608–249–0487

Wyoming Division, Inc.
2222 House Avenue
Cheyenne, Wyoming 82001
307–638–3331

CANCER CARE, INC.
1180 Avenue of the Americas
New York, New York 10036
212–221–3300

The service arm of the National Cancer Foundation, which provides information, counseling, and support for patients and family members.

CANDLELIGHTERS CHILDHOOD CANCER FOUNDATION, INC.
1901 Pennsylvania Avenue N.W.
Washington, D.C. 20006
202–659–5136

An international organization of parents whose children have or have had cancer. The society provides guidance and support services.

CONCERN FOR DYING
250 West 57th Street
New York, New York 10107
212–246–6962

An educational organization that distributes information on the Living Will, a document that records patient wishes on medical treatment, death, and dying.

CORPORATE ANGEL NETWORK
Westchester County Airport
Hangar F
White Plains, New York 10604
914–328–1313

An organization to alleviate the costs of cancer patients undergoing therapy in National Cancer Institute–approved centers by arranging free transportation on corporate aircraft.

LEUKEMIA SOCIETY OF AMERICA, INC.
733 Third Avenue
New York, New York 10017
212–573–8484

A national organization that supports research on leukemia and provides consultation and financial assistance for patients with leukemia and related diseases.

MAKE-A-WISH FOUNDATION OF AMERICA
2600 North Central Avenue, Suite 936
Phoenix, Arizona 85004
602–240–6600

An organization to cover expenses and arrange for granting a "special wish" for terminally ill children.

MAKE TODAY COUNT
101/2 South Union Street
Alexandria, Virginia 22314
703–548–9674

An association of cancer patients and other people with life-threatening diseases, family members, nurses, physicians, and community members. The organization provides emotional self-help.

NATIONAL CANCER INSTITUTE
National Institutes of Health
Bethesda, Maryland 20892

The National Cancer Institute is the division of the National Institutes of Health that supports programs of cancer research and treatment, as well as providing a variety of information services to patients and physicians.

Cancer Information Service
800–4–CANCER

A toll-free number by which patients or family members are connected to staff members trained to answer a variety of questions about cancer.

Office of Cancer Communications
National Cancer Institute
Building 31, Room 10A24
Bethesda, Maryland 20892

This office provides a wide variety of written materials on cancer for both patients and physicians.

PDQ (Physician Data Query) Service

A computerized database providing current treatment information for most types of cancer, descriptions of ongoing clinical trials, and names of organizations and physicians involved in cancer treatment. The Cancer Information Service (800–4–CANCER) provides free PDQ searches.

NCI Comprehensive Cancer Centers

Comprehensive cancer centers are National Cancer Institute–recognized centers for cancer research and treatment.

Alabama
University of Alabama
Comprehensive Cancer Center
205–934–5077

California
Kenneth Norris, Jr., Comprehensive
  Cancer Center
University of Southern California
213–224–6600

Jonsson Comprehensive Cancer Center
University of California at Los Angeles
213–825–3181

Connecticut
Yale University Comprehensive
  Cancer Center
203–785–4095

Florida
Sylvester Comprehensive Cancer
  Center
University of Miami
305–548–4800

Illinois
Illinois Cancer Council
312–346–9813

Maryland
Johns Hopkins Oncology Center
301–955–8822

Massachusetts
Dana-Farber Cancer Institute
617–732–3000

Michigan
Comprehensive Cancer Center
Wayne State University
313–745–8870

Minnesota
Mayo Comprehensive Cancer Center
507–284–4718

New York
Columbia University Cancer Center
212–305–6921

Memorial Sloan-Kettering Cancer
  Center
212–639–6561

Roswell Park Memorial Institute
716–845–5770

North Carolina
Duke Comprehensive Cancer Center
919–684–3377

Lineberger Cancer Research Center
University of North Carolina
919–966–3036

Cancer Center
Bowman Gray School of Medicine
Wake Forest University
919–748–4464

Ohio
Comprehensive Cancer Center
Ohio State University
614–293–3302

Pennsylvania
Fox Chase Cancer Center
215–728–2781

Pittsburgh Cancer Institute
University of Pittsburgh
412–647–2072

Texas
M.D. Anderson Cancer Center
University of Texas
713–792–6000

Washington
Fred Hutchinson Cancer Research
   Center
206–467–4302

Wisconsin
Clinical Cancer Center
University of Wisconsin
608–263–8610

NATIONAL COALITION FOR CANCER SURVIVORSHIP
323 8th Street S.W.
Albuquerque, New Mexico 87102
505–764–9956

A network of groups concerned with the issues facing cancer survivors.

NATIONAL HOSPICE ORGANIZATION
1901 North Fort Myer Drive, Suite 901
Arlington, Virginia 22209
703–243–5900

An organization of groups and institutions dealing with care for the terminally ill and their families. The organization provides information and referrals.

UNITED OSTOMY ASSOCIATION, INC.
36 Executive Park, Suite 120
Irvine, California 92714
714–660–8624

The association provides counseling and support for patients who have had colostomy, ileostomy, or urostomy surgery.

Glossary

abl   An oncogene involved in chronic myelogenous and acute lymphocytic leukemias.

Actinomycin D   A chemotherapeutic drug that binds to DNA and inhibits RNA synthesis.

Acute lymphocytic leukemia (ALL)   A rapidly progressing leukemia of immature lymphocytes.

Acute monocytic leukemia   A rapidly progressing leukemia of immature monocytes.

Acute myelocytic leukemia (AML)   A rapidly progressing leukemia of myeloblastic cells (immature granulocytes).

Acute myelomonocytic leukemia   A rapidly progressing leukemia of precursors to both granulocytes and monocytes.

Acute promyelocytic leukemia (APL)   A rapidly progressing leukemia of promyelocytes (granulocyte precursors).

Adenocarcinoma   A cancer arising from glandular epithelium.

Adenoma   A benign tumor arising from glandular epithelium.

Aflatoxin   A potent liver carcinogen found in contaminated food supplies.

Alkylating agents   A group of chemotherapeutic drugs that react with DNA.

Androgen   A steroid hormone that stimulates male sex characteristics.

Angiography   X-ray examination of the blood vessels.

Antibody   A protein secreted by B lymphocytes that recognizes foreign substances.

Antimetabolite   A chemotherapeutic drug that interferes with one or more steps in DNA synthesis.

APC   A tumor suppressor gene involved in colon cancers.

Asparaginase   An enzyme used in chemotherapy that degrades the amino acid asparagine.

Astrocytoma   A type of malignant brain tumor.

Ataxia telangiectasia   An inherited disease associated with genetic instability, immunodeficiency, and an increased susceptibility to leukemias and lymphomas.

Basal cell carcinoma   A common type of skin cancer.

B cell   See B lymphocyte.

bcl-2   An oncogene involved in follicular B-cell lymphomas that acts by inhibiting cell death.

Benign tumor   A tumor that remains confined to its original location and does not invade adjacent tissue or metastasize to distant body sites.

Bischloroethylnitrosourea (BCNU)   An alkylating agent used in chemotherapy.

Bleomycin   A chemotherapeutic drug that reacts with DNA.

Blocking agent   A chemopreventive drug that interferes with the action of carcinogens.

Bloom's syndrome   An inherited disease associated with genetic instability and an increased incidence of leukemias and lymphomas.

B lymphocyte   An antibody-producing lymphocyte.

Bone marrow transplantation   A procedure in which patients receive high doses of chemotherapeutic drugs or radiation, followed by a transplant of new bone marrow to bypass toxicity to the blood-forming cells.

Burkitt's lymphoma   A non-Hodgkin's B-cell lymphoma associated with Epstein-Barr virus infection.

CA-125   A tumor marker for ovarian carcinomas.

Cancer   A malignant tumor.

Carcinoembryonic antigen (CEA)   A tumor marker frequently secreted by gastrointestinal carcinomas.

Carcinogen   A cancer-inducing agent.

Carcinogenesis   Development of cancer.

Carcinoma   A malignant tumor of epithelial cells.

Carcinoma *in situ*   A small carcinoma that has not yet invaded surrounding normal tissue.

Cells   The smallest living structures, of which all living things are composed.

Chemoprevention   The administration of drugs to reduce cancer risk.

Chemotherapy   The treatment of cancer with drugs.

Chlorambucil   An alkylating agent used in chemotherapy.

Choriocarcinoma   A type of cancer arising from male or female germ cells.

Chromosome   A DNA molecule associated with proteins in the cell nucleus.

Chronic lymphocytic leukemia (CLL)   A slowly progressing leukemia of immature lymphocytes.

Chronic myelogenous leukemia (CML)   A slowly progressing leukemia originating in the pluripotent stem cell of the bone marrow.

Cirrhosis   A disease characterized by liver-cell degeneration.

Cisplatin   A platinum compound used in chemotherapy.

Clinical staging   See tumor staging.

Clinical trial   Testing of new drugs in cancer patients.

Colonoscopy   Examination of the colon with a flexible, lighted tube.

Combination chemotherapy   The use of drug combinations for cancer treatment.

Computed tomography (CT or CAT) scan   A scanning x-ray technique that employs computer analysis to generate cross-sectional images of the body.

Contact inhibition   The cessation of movement of normal cells that results from contact with other cells.

Cruciferous vegetables   The group of vegetables, including broccoli, Brussels sprouts, and cauliflower, that contain several compounds inhibiting cancer development.

Cyclohexylchloroethylnitrosourea (CCNU)   An alkylating agent used in chemotherapy.

Cyclophosphamide   An alkylating agent used in chemotherapy.

Cystoscopy   Examination of the bladder with a thin, lighted tube.

Cytosine arabinoside   An antimetabolite that inhibits DNA replication.

Daunomycin   A chemotherapeutic drug that binds to and damages DNA.

DCC   A tumor suppressor gene involved in colon and rectum cancers.

Diethylstilbestrol (DES)   A synthetic estrogen.

DNA   Deoxyribonucleic acid; the genetic material.

Doxorubicin   A chemotherapeutic drug that binds to and damages DNA.

Drug resistance   Failure of cancer cells to respond to a chemotherapeutic drug.

Ductal carcinoma   A type of breast cancer that arises in the ducts of the mammary gland.

Dysgerminoma   An ovarian tumor of undifferentiated germ cells.

Dysplasia   An early, preneoplastic stage of the development of carcinomas characterized by loss of cellular regularity.

Embryonal carcinoma   A cancer of embryonic cells.

Endometrium   The lining of the uterus.

Endoscopy   The use of thin, lighted tubes for examination of internal body cavities.

Ependymoma   A type of malignant brain tumor.

Epidemiology   Study of the incidence of disease in different population groups.

Epithelial cells   Cells that form continuous sheets covering the surface of the body and lining the internal organs.

Epstein-Barr virus   A virus associated with Burkitt's lymphoma and nasopharyngeal carcinoma.

*erb*B-2   An oncogene involved in breast and ovarian carcinomas.

Erythrocyte   Red blood cell.

Erythroleukemia   A leukemia of immature red blood cells.

Estrogen   A steroid hormone that stimulates female sex characteristics.

Estrogen replacement therapy   Administration of estrogen to relieve symptoms of menopause.

Etoposide   A chemotherapeutic drug that causes DNA breakage.

Ewing's sarcoma   A childhood bone tumor.

Familial adenomatous polyposis   A rare, inherited form of colon cancer in which affected individuals develop multiple colon adenomas (polyps).

Fanconi's anemia   A hereditary disease characterized by genetic instability and a high incidence of leukemias and lymphomas.

Fecal occult blood test   A colon cancer screening test in which the presence of small amounts of blood in the stool is detected.

Fluorouracil   An antimetabolite that inhibits DNA replication.

Gastroscopy   Examination of the stomach with a thin, lighted tube.

Gene   The basic unit of heredity; a region of DNA that encodes a single protein.

Genome   The complete genetic information of a species.

Glioblastoma   A highly malignant type of astrocytoma.

Glioma   Any brain tumor arising from glial (supporting) cells. (Astrocytomas are a type of glioma.)

Gonadotropin   A hormone produced by the pituitary that controls the function of the gonads.

Gonadotropin-releasing hormone (GnRH)   A hormone produced by the hypothalamus that acts on the pituitary to signal gonadotropin release.

Grading   See tumor grading.

Graft-versus-host disease   The principal complication of bone marrow transplantation, in which lymphocytes from the donor marrow react against cells of the recipient.

Granulocyte   A type of white blood cell that functions in inflammation.

Growth factor   A secreted protein that stimulates cell division.

Growth-factor receptor   A cell surface protein to which a growth factor binds.

Hepatitis B viruses   A family of viruses that can cause liver cancer.

Hodgkin's disease   A type of lymphoma.

Hormone   A chemical produced by one type of cell that affects the activity of a second type of cell.

Hospice   An organization designed to provide care for terminally ill patients.

Human immunodeficiency virus (HIV)   The virus that causes AIDS.

Human T-cell lymphotropic virus (HTLV)   A virus that causes adult T-cell leukemia.

Hydroxyurea   A chemotherapeutic drug that inhibits DNA replication.

Imaging   The use of noninvasive methods, such as x-rays, to view the inside of the body.

Immune system   The body's defense against infection.

Immunosuppressive   Suppressing the activity of the immune system.

Immunotherapy   Stimulating the immune system to eliminate cancer cells.

Inflammatory carcinoma   A type of breast cancer.

Interferon   A secreted factor that inhibits virus infection and displays antitumor activity.

Interleukin-2 (IL-2)   A growth factor that stimulates proliferation of T lymphocytes.

Ionizing radiation   High energy forms of radiation, such as x-rays and radiation produced by the decay of radioactive particles.

Kaposi's sarcoma   A vascular tumor common in AIDS patients.

Leukemia   A cancer arising from the blood-forming cells in bone marrow.

Levamisole   A nonspecific immune stimulant used in tumor therapy.

Li-Fraumeni cancer family syndrome   A rare, hereditary cancer susceptibility, leading to the development of multiple kinds of tumors, which results from inherited mutations of the *p53* tumor suppressor gene.

Lobular carcinoma   A type of breast cancer that arises in the lobules of the mammary gland.

Lymphatic system   The structural system involved in the immune response, which includes lymphatic vessels, lymph nodes, spleen, tonsils, and thymus.

Lymph node   An aggregate of lymphatic tissue.

Lymphocyte   A white blood cell that functions in the immune response.

Lymphoid   The blood-cell lineage giving rise to lymphocytes.

Lymphoma   A cancer arising from lymphocytes or macrophages in lymphatic tissue.

Lynch cancer family syndrome   A rare, inherited cancer susceptibility leading to the development of breast and ovarian carcinomas.

Macrophage   A white blood cell that functions in inflammatory reactions and the immune response.

Magnetic resonance imaging (MRI)   An imaging technique that employs computer analysis of the movement of molecules in a strong magnetic field.

Malignant tumor   A tumor that is capable of invading surrounding normal tissue and metastasizing to distant body sites.

Mammogram   A low-dose x-ray of the breast.

MCC   A tumor suppressor gene involved in colon and rectum carcinomas.

Mechlorethamine   Nitrogen mustard; an alkylating agent used in chemotherapy.

Medulloblastoma   A type of malignant brain tumor most common in children.

Melanoma   A cancer of the pigment-producing cells of the skin.

Melphalan   An alkylating agent used in chemotherapy.

Meningioma   A type of benign brain tumor.

Mercaptopurine   An antimetabolite that inhibits DNA replication.

Metastasis   The spread of cancer cells to distant body sites.

Methotrexate   An antimetabolite that interferes with DNA replication.

Mitomycin C   A chemotherapeutic drug that reacts with DNA.

Monoclonal antibody   An antibody, directed against a unique target, that is produced by a single clone of B lymphocytes.

Monocyte   A type of white blood cell involved in inflammatory reactions.

Multidrug resistance   Simultaneous resistance of a tumor to multiple chemotherapeutic drugs.

Multiple myeloma   Cancer of mature antibody-producing B lymphocytes (plasma cells).

Mutagen   An agent that induces mutations.

Mutation   An alteration in the base sequence of DNA.

myc   A family of oncogenes (c-*myc*, L-*myc*, and N-*myc*) which are involved in a variety of tumors, including Burkitt's and other B-cell lymphomas, neuroblastomas, and small-cell lung carcinomas.

Myeloid   The blood-cell lineage giving rise to platelets, erythrocytes, granulocytes, monocytes, and macrophages.

Neoplasm   An abnormal growth of cells.

Neuroblastoma   A childhood cancer of embryonic neural cells.

Neurofibroma   A benign tumor arising from connective tissue of a nerve.

NF1   A tumor suppressor gene responsible for inheritance of type 1(von Recklinghausen) neurofibromatosis.

Nitrogen mustard   An alkylating agent used in chemotherapy.

Nitrosamines   A class of carcinogens that can be formed from nitrates and nitrites in the digestive tract.

Non-Hodgkin's lymphoma   Any type of lymphoma other than Hodgkin's disease.

Nuclear magnetic resonance (NMR)   See Magnetic resonance imaging.

Occupational carcinogen   A carcinogen to which workers are exposed.

Oncogene   A gene capable of inducing one or more characteristics of cancer cells.

Ostomy   A surgical procedure that creates a new opening to the surface of the body.

Osteosarcoma   A type of bone tumor.

p53   A tumor suppressor gene involved in a wide variety of cancers, including breast, colon, and lung carcinomas, sarcomas, and leukemias.

Pap test   A screening test for early detection of cervical carcinoma.

Papilloma   A benign tumor projecting from a surface.

Papillomaviruses   A family of tumor viruses that induce papillomas and carcinomas in a variety of species, including anogenital carcinomas in humans.

Philadelphia chromosome An abnormal human chromosome 22, formed by translocation of the *abl* oncogene from chromosome 9 in chronic myelogenous leukemias.

Platelet A blood cell that functions in coagulation.

Platelet-derived growth factor (PDGF) A growth factor that stimulates proliferation of connective tissue cells.

Polyp A benign tumor projecting from a surface.

Prednisone A hormone used in treatment of leukemias and lymphomas.

Premalignant A neoplastic cell that has not yet acquired the ability to invade surrounding normal tissue.

Preneoplastic A cell that displays increased proliferative potential and is capable of progressing to the full neoplastic phenotype as a result of further alterations.

Procarbazine An alkylating agent used in chemotherapy.

Progesterone A steroid hormone secreted by the corpus luteum that functions to prepare the uterine endometrium for implantation of a developing embryo.

Promoting agent A compound that leads to tumor development by stimulating cell proliferation.

Prostate-specific antigen (PSA) A protein secreted by prostate cells which is a marker for prostate carcinoma.

Protein The product encoded by a gene.

Radioisotope scanning An imaging method in which radioactive isotopes are administered and then detected in tissues of the patient.

Radon A natural source of radiation formed as a decay product of uranium.

RAR The retinoic-acid receptor, which is mutated to act as an oncogene in acute promyelocytic leukemia.

ras A family of oncogenes (*ras*H, *ras*K, and *ras*N) involved in a variety of human tumors, including colon, lung, pancreatic, and thyroid carcinomas, leukemias, and lymphomas.

RB A tumor suppressor gene identified by genetic studies of retinoblastoma, and also involved in osteosarcomas, rhabdomyosarcomas, and bladder, breast, lung, and prostate carcinomas.

Reed-Sternberg cell   The characteristic cell of Hodgkin's disease.

Retinoblastoma   A childhood eye tumor.

Retinoic acid (vitamin A)   A hormone that induces differentiation and inhibits proliferation of a variety of cell types.

Retinoids   Compounds related to retinoic acid.

Rhabdomyosarcoma   A cancer of skeletal muscle cells.

Risk factor   A factor affecting the likelihood that an individual will develop cancer.

RNA   Ribonucleic acid; the chemical messenger that carries information from DNA out to the cytoplasm to direct protein synthesis.

Sarcoma   A cancer of connective tissue.

Screening   Testing to detect early stages of cancer development in healthy, asymptomatic individuals.

Secondary prevention   Screening to detect early stages of cancer development that are readily treatable.

Seminoma   A cancer of undifferentiated germ cells.

Sigmoidoscopy   Endoscopic examination of the rectum and lower part of the colon.

Small cell carcinoma   A type of lung cancer.

Squamous cell carcinoma   A cancer of flat epithelial cells.

Staging   See tumor staging.

Steroid hormones   A group of hormones, including estrogens, androgens, progesterone, glucocorticoids, thyroid hormone, and retinoic acid.

Suppressing agent   A chemopreventive agent that acts to inhibit cell proliferation.

Tamoxifen   An estrogen antagonist.

Taxol   A chemotherapeutic drug that blocks cell division.

T cell   See T lymphocyte.

Teniposide   A chemotherapeutic drug that causes DNA breakage.

Teratoma   A tumor of embryonic cells.

Testosterone   A steroid hormone produced by the testes that stimulates male sex characteristics.

Thioguanine An antimetabolite that inhibits DNA replication.

Thiotepa An alkylating agent used in chemotherapy.

T lymphocyte A lymphocyte that functions in cell-mediated immune responses.

TNM system A system of tumor staging based on tumor size, invasion of surrounding tissue, lymph node involvement, and metastasis.

Transitional cell carcinoma A carcinoma arising from the transitional epithelium of the bladder.

Tumor An abnormal growth of cells.

Tumor grading Histologic (microscopic) examination of tumor cell morphology and rate of cell division.

Tumor-infiltrating lymphocyte (TIL) A lymphocyte with antitumor activity.

Tumor initiation The first step in development of a tumor.

Tumor marker A substance, produced by cancer cells, that can be used as a diagnostic test for tumor growth.

Tumor necrosis factor (TNF) A secreted factor with antitumor activity.

Tumor progression The continuing development of increasing malignancy during growth of a tumor.

Tumor promoter A compound that leads to tumor development by stimulating cell proliferation.

Tumor staging Assessment of the extent of tumor growth, invasion, and metastasis.

Tumor suppressor gene A gene that inhibits tumor development.

Ultrasonography An imaging method in which the echoes of high-frequency sound waves are used to reveal tissue masses.

Vinblastine A chemotherapeutic drug that blocks cell division.

Vincristine A chemotherapeutic drug that blocks cell division.

Virus An infectious particle that reproduces inside cells.

VP-16 See etoposide.

Warthin cancer family syndrome A rare, inherited cancer susceptibility leading to the development of colon and endometrial cancers.

Wilms' tumor   A childhood kidney cancer.

WT1   A tumor suppressor gene involved in Wilms' tumor.

Xeroderma pigmentosum   An inherited skin disease, associated with a high incidence of skin cancer, in which patients are unable to repair DNA damage resulting from ultraviolet light.

Yolk sac carcinoma   A type of embryonic tumor arising from male or female germ cells.

Further Reading

GENERAL BOOKS AND REFERENCES

American Cancer Society. 1992. *Cancer Facts and Figures 1992*. Atlanta: American Cancer Society.

Dollinger, M., Rosenbaum, E. H., and Cable, G. 1991. *Everyone's Guide to Cancer Therapy*. Toronto: Somerville House Books.

Kubler-Ross, E. 1969. *On Death and Dying*. New York: Macmillan.

Laszlo, J. 1987. *Understanding Cancer*. New York: Harper & Row.

Love, S. 1990. *Dr. Susan Love's Breast Book*. Reading, MA: Addison-Wesley.

Morra, M., and Potts, E. 1987. *Choices: Realistic Alternatives in Cancer Treatment*. New York: Avon Books.

National Research Council. 1989. *Diet and Health: Implications for Reducing Chronic Disease Risk*. Washington D.C.: National Academy Press.

Nero, A. V., Jr. 1988. Controlling indoor air pollution. *Scientific American* 258:42–48.

Nessim, S., and Ellis, J. 1991. *Cancervive: The Challenge of Life after Cancer*. Boston: Houghton Mifflin.

Page, H. S., and Asire, A. J. 1985. *Cancer Rates and Risks* (3rd ed). Bethesda, MD: National Institutes of Health.

U.S. Congress, Office of Technology Assessment. 1990. *Unconventional Cancer Treatments*. Washington D.C.: U.S. Government Printing Office.

U.S. Dept. of Health and Human Services. 1989. Reducing the Health Consequences of Smoking: 25 Years of Progress. A Report of the Surgeon General.

U.S. Dept. of Health and Human Services. 1992. *Healthy People 2000: National Health Promotion and Disease Prevention Objectives*. Boston: Jones and Bartlett.

MEDICAL AND SCIENTIFIC BOOKS

Brugge, J., Curran, T., Harlow, E., and McCormick, F. (eds.) 1991. *Origins of Human Cancer: A Comprehensive Review*. Cold Spring Harbor, NY: Cold Spring Harbor Laboratory Press.

Cairns, J. 1978. *Cancer: Science and Society*. New York: Freeman.

Chabner, B. A., and Collins, J. M. (eds.) 1990. *Cancer Chemotherapy: Principles and Practice*. Philadelphia: Lippincott.

Cooper, G. M. 1992. *Elements of Human Cancer*. Boston: Jones and Bartlett.

Cooper, G. M. 1990. *Oncogenes*. Boston: Jones and Bartlett.

DeVita, V. T., Jr., Hellman, S., and Rosenberg, S.A. (eds.) 1989. *Cancer: Principles and Practice of Oncology* (3rd ed.) Philadelphia: Lippincott.

Doll, R., and Peto, R. 1981. *The Causes of Cancer*. New York: Oxford University Press.

Groenwald, S. L., Frogge, M. H., Goodman, M., and Yarbro, C. H. 1993. *Cancer Nursing: Principles and Practice* (3rd ed.). Boston: Jones and Bartlett.

Jandl, J. H. 1991. *Blood: Pathophysiology*. Boston: Blackwell Scientific Publications.

Kupchella, C. E. 1987. *Dimensions of Cancer*. Belmont, CA: Wadsworth.

Pitot, H. C. 1986. *Fundamentals of Oncology* (3rd ed.). New York: Marcel Dekker.

Prescott, D. M., and Flexer, A. S. 1986. *Cancer: The Misguided Cell* (2nd ed.). Sunderland, MA: Sinauer Associates.

Ruddon, R. W. 1987. *Cancer Biology* (2nd ed.). New York: Oxford University Press.

SELECTED ARTICLES IN MEDICAL AND SCIENTIFIC JOURNALS

Aaronson, S. A. 1991. Growth factors and cancer. *Science* 254:1146–1153.

Ames, B. N., and Gold, L. S. 1990. Too many rodent carcinogens: Mitogenesis increases mutagenesis. *Science* 249:970–971.

Bishop, J. M. 1991. Molecular themes in oncogenesis. *Cell* 64:235–248.

Black, P. M. 1991. Brain tumors (two parts). *New England Journal of Medicine* 324:1471–1476 and 1555–1564.

Bonadonna, G. 1992. Evolving concepts in the systemic adjuvant treatment of breast cancer. *Cancer Research* 52:2127–2137.

Cannon-Albright, L. A., Skolnick, M. H., Bishop, D. T., Lee, R. G., and Burt, R. W. 1988. Common inheritance of susceptibility to colonic adenomatous polyps and associated colorectal cancers. *New England Journal of Medicine* 319:533–537.

Castiagne, S., Chomienne, C., Daniel, M. T., Ballerini, P., Berger, R., Fenaux, P., and Degos, L. 1990. All-trans retinoic acid as a differentiation therapy for acute promyelocytic leukemia. I. Clinical results. *Blood* 76:1704–1709.

Castonguay, A. 1992. Methods and strategies in lung cancer control. *Cancer Research* 52:2641s–2651s.

Catalona, W. J., Smith, D. S., Ratliff, T. L., Dodds, K. M., Coplen, D. E., Yuan, J. J. J., Petros, J. A., and Andriole, G. L. 1991. Measurement of prostate-specific antigen in serum as a screening test for prostate cancer. *New England Journal of Medicine* 324:1156–1161.

Crist, W. M., and Kun, L. E. 1991. Common solid tumors of childhood. *New England Journal of Medicine* 324:461–471.

Eddy, D. M. 1990. Screening for cervical cancer. *Annals of Internal Medicine* 113:214–226.

Fearon, E., and Vogelstein, B. 1990. A genetic model for colorectal tumorigenesis. *Cell* 61:759–767.

Fisher, B. 1992. The evolution of paradigms for the management of breast cancer: A personal perspective. *Cancer Research* 52:2371–2383.

Ganz, P. A. 1992. Treatment options for breast cancer—Beyond survival. *New England Journal of Medicine* 326:1147–1149.

Gittes, R. F. 1991. Carcinoma of the prostate. *New England Journal of Medicine* 324:236–245.

Harris, J. R., Lippman, M. E., Veronesi, U. and Willett, W. 1992. Breast cancer (three parts). *New England Journal of Medicine* 327:319–328, 390–398, and 473–480.

Henderson, B. E., Ross, R., and Bernstein, L. 1988. Estrogens as a cause of human cancer. *Cancer Research* 48:246–253.

Henderson, B. E., Ross, R. K., and Pike, M. C. 1991. Towards the primary prevention of cancer. *Science* 254:1131–1138.

Hollstein, M., Sidransky, D., Vogelstein, B., and Harris, C. C. 1991. *p53* mutations in human cancers. *Science* 253:49–53.

Jackson, J. D. 1992. Are the stray 60-Hz electromagnetic fields associated with the distribution and use of electric power a significant cause of cancer? *Proceedings of the National Academy of Sciences USA* 89:3508–3510.

Knudson, A. G., Jr. 1985. Genetics of human cancer. *Annual Review of Genetics* 20:231–251.

Kyle, R. A. 1990. Newer approaches to the therapy of multiple myeloma. *Blood* 76:1678–1679.

Levin, B. 1992. Screening sigmoidoscopy for colorectal cancer. *New England Journal of Medicine* 326:700–702.

Link, M. P., Donaldson, S. S., Berard, C. W., Shuster, J. J., and Murphy, S. B. 1990. Results of treatment of childhood localized non-Hodgkin's lymphoma with combination chemotherapy with or without radiotherapy. *New England Journal of Medicine* 322:1169–1174.

Look, A. T., Hayes, F. A., Shuster, J. J., Douglass, E. C., Castleberry, R. P., Bowman, L. C., Smith, E. I., and Brodeur, G. M. 1991. Clinical relevance of tumor cell ploidy and N-*myc* gene amplification in childhood neuroblastoma. *Journal of Clinical Oncology* 9:581–591.

Meyskens, F. L., Jr. 1990. Coming of age—The chemoprevention of cancer. *New England Journal of Medicine* 323:825–827.

Moertel, C. G., Fleming, T. R., MacDonald, J. S., Haller, D. G., Laurie, J. A., Goodman, P. J., Underleider, J. S., Emerson, W. A., Tormey, D. C., Glick, J. H., Veeder, M. H., and Mailliard, J. A. 1990. Levamisole and fluorouracil for adjuvant therapy of resected colon carcinoma. *New England Journal of Medicine* 322:352–358.

Mulvihill, J. J. 1985. Clinical ecogenetics: Cancer in families. *New England Journal of Medicine* 312:1569–1570.

Pastan, I., and Gottesman, M. 1987. Multiple-drug resistance in human cancer. *New England Journal of Medicine* 316:1388–1393.

Preston-Martin, S., Pike, M. C., Ross, R. K., Jones, P. A., and Henderson, B. E. 1990. Increased cell division as a cause of human cancer. *Cancer Research* 50:7415–7421.

Raghavan, D., Shipley, W. U., Garnick, M. B., Russell, P. J., and Richie, J. P. 1990. Biology and management of bladder cancer. *New England Journal of Medicine* 322:1129–1138.

Rivera, G. K., Raimondi, S. C., Hancock, M. L., Behm, F. G., Pui, C. H., Abromowitch, M., Mirro, J., Jr., Ochs, J. S., Look, A. T., Williams, D. T., Murphy, S. B., Dahl, G. V., Kalwinsky, D. K., Evans, W. E., Kun, L. E., Simone, J. V., and Crist, W. M. 1991. Improved outcome in childhood acute lymphoblastic leukaemia with reinforced early treatment and rotational combination chemotherapy. *Lancet* 337:61–66.

Roth, J. A. 1992. New approaches to treating early lung cancer. *Cancer Research* 52:2652s–2657s.

Shapiro, S. 1989. The status of breast cancer screening: A quarter-century of research. *World Journal of Surgery* 13:9–18.

Skolnick, M. H., Cannon-Albright, L. A., Goldgar, D. E., Ward, J. H., Marshall, C. J., Schumann, G. B., Hogle, H., McWhorter, W. P., Wright, E. C., Tran, T. D., Bishop, D. T., Kushner, J. P., and Eyre, H. J. 1990. Inheritance of proliferative breast disease in breast cancer. *Science* 250:1715–1720.

Solomon, E., Borrow, J., and Goddard, A. D. 1991. Chromosome aberrations and cancer. *Science* 254:1153–1160.

Tobias, J. S. 1992. Clinical practice of radiotherapy. *Lancet* 339:159–163.

Vedantham, S., Gamliel, H., and Golomb, H. M. 1992. Mechanism of interferon action in hairy cell leukemia: A model of effective cancer biotherapy. *Cancer Research* 52:1056–1066.

Voigt, L. F., Weiss, N. S., Chu, J., Daling, J. R., McKnight, B., and van Belle, G. 1991. Progestagen supplementation of exogenous oestrogens and risk of endometrial cancer. *Lancet* 338:274–277.

Warshaw, A. L., and Fernandez-del Castillo, C. 1992. Pancreatic carcinoma. *New England Journal of Medicine* 326:455–465.

Weinberg, R. A. 1991. Tumor suppressor genes. *Science* 254:1138–1146.

Willett, W. 1989. The search for the causes of breast and colon cancer. *Nature* 338:389–394.

Willett, W. C., Stampfer, M. J., Colditz, G. A., Rosner, B. A., and Speizer, F. E. 1990. Relation of meat, fat, and fiber intake to the risk of colon cancer in a prospective study among women. *New England Journal of Medicine* 323:1664–1672.

Zur Hausen, H. 1991. Viruses in human cancer. *Science* 254:1167–1173.

Index

continued

continued